Finding Joy in the Everyday

A Journey of Grief and Gratitude

Susanna Lewis

Starry Skies Publishing

Published by Starry Skies Publishing.

Cover Design by Edwin Rydberg at Quantum Dot Press www.quantumdotpress.com

Contents

DEDICATION

This book is dedicated to my lovely, and much missed Mum. She taught me to write and to believe in the magic of storytelling.

And I would also like to say thank you to both my Mum and Dad for always being part of my life and always supporting me through the good and bad times. I miss you both so much, but will love you forever.

Chapter One

My Story

My journey starts in an unusual place. March 2023 to be exact. In fact, this book starts three days after the funeral of my beloved mother, the end of her life, the beginning of a new and unknown life for me. A complicated, deep dive into the world of grief, loss and confusion, a place most of us will visit at some time in our life.

For many years I was my Mum's carer as she battled through the soul sapping illness, that we know as dementia. This cruel and unpredictable affliction changed my Mum's life beyond recognition, but it also changed mine. I was thrust into an unknown world, trying to find my way through the confusion and angst, without directions or even a roadmap on how to navigate the muddy waters of this sad and lonely journey. Mum and I battled through Covid together. As the world shut down, so did my Mum. Without any support from the medical professionals, I focused my thoughts on just keeping her alive during the pandemic. It was, without doubt, the most difficult time of my life. The woman that I loved unconditionally now relied on me for her care and wellbeing. The mother became the daughter and the daughter became the mother. Of course, it was a privilege to care for her, to repay her for all that she had done for me, but it was a huge relief when, she finally was admitted to a care home, a place where she would be safe and cared for 24/7.

After a difficult few months in late 2022 and early 2023, my lovely Mum passed away in late February 2023. The pain and grief was so intense that it took me completely by surprise. My life as a carer and daughter was over and I struggled to accept my new life, without Mum. And so, I turned to writing. Writing has always been a constant in my life, whether I am writing cosy crime fiction or heartfelt poetry. Words have the power to help us through difficult stages of our life, comforting our emotions and soothing our tired minds. I have such a deep and profound love for writing that it feels an integral part of my world. It was therefore inevitable that I would use writing to help me through the grief and loss, following Mum's passing.

I am a prolific journaller. I write and photograph about my daily life and my observations of the world as I see them. I note down conversations I overhear, the colour of spring flowers I see on my daily walk, the taste of creamy coffee as it dances around my mouth and the smell of a fresh, warm croissant. I use my journal as a way of practicing mindfulness, to help calm an often busy and cluttered mind. I am a trained therapeutic and reflective writing teacher, and I see so many ordinary people benefitting from the power of writing and journalling. It truly is wonderful to see how the magic of putting words on paper can bring peace to the writer.

I am also an advocate of gratitude journalling. Every evening, after I have completed writing my journal entries, I also write down three things of the day that I am truly grateful for, however small they may be. Gratitude journalling can give us a profound sense of appreciation of the world in which we live, and I believe it also has the power to transform our mood to a more positive one. At the end of each chapter in this book you will find my own personal gratitude entries for that particular day. I hope you enjoy reading them, and maybe it might encourage you to start your own gratitude journal. If you do, please let me know how you get on.

This book is a reflection of twelve months of my life from March 2023 through to the end of February 2024, with entries taken from my journal. I chose this particular period in my life as my mother had passed away in February 2023 and I needed my journalling more than ever to get me through this difficult time. Each chapter records my observations of life on a particular day. I have used selected days for the purpose of this book, to try and give you, the reader, a snapshot of my life over the twelve months. I have captured real life events, conversations and observations, including my own personal dark moments, but interspersed with humour and hopefulness.

Grief is different for everyone, and we each get through it the best way we can. I chose to increase my mindful activities by recording daily observations in my notebook, and I felt this helped the deep, piercing feeling of loss, the emptiness caused by my mother's passing. Focusing on random conversations and everyday real life situations helped me move away from the raw grief that was impacting on my life. It was my way of coping with the sad feelings. It was a way of finding joy in the simplest of things.

And so this book starts on the 20th March 2023, the first day of spring and just three days after the funeral.

I hope you enjoy the quirky observations, the feelings and emotions, the 'little things' that make us smile and make us feel alive. And if you too are going through grief, then I hope you find a way to manage your own feelings, and please know that you have my support and love as you travel on this difficult journey.

With love

Susanna x

Chapter Two

Monday 20th March 2023

Today is the first day of spring. Remnants of Mum's funeral lie scattered around the house. Wilting coffee coloured daffodils bow their heads with exhaustion, much like myself. Sympathy cards adorn the windowsill, each one a reminder of the love and support I have felt over the last few weeks. Gazing into the garden I see delicate green buds unfurling on the barren tree, excited to wake from their winter slumber. I also start to unfurl, stretching out into a new world, a world without Mum.

It is Monday and as the world starts a new working week, I cautiously leave the house, feeling empty, but resolving to embrace life, as Mum would have wished. The deep seated pain that lies heavy on my chest follows me as I shut the front door behind me, my dog George eagerly pulling on his lead.

Just one step at a time Susanna. Let's do this.

***

My dog George, stops to sniff at the corner of my neighbour's garden wall. I watch him as he excitedly wags his tail and I wonder what type of dog stopped there this morning. What was their name? What does their owner look like? Are they suffering with grief too? My thought pattern is interrupted as my neighbour comes out just as George pees on his wall. I am mortified and offer a weak, pathetic smile. I'm guessing there will be no neighbourly Christmas card this year.

***

An elderly man walks towards me, supported by a rather old fashioned walking stick. I hear the 'tap tap' of the wooden cane as he edges closer to me and I wonder if he knows how loud the sound is. He nods at me.

'Good morning. Lovely day'

I smile back, trying to ignore the fact that it is raining.

'Good morning.'

***

In the churchyard there are more wilting daffodils, bowing their heads, tired of life. It's a sign that matches my mood. Still, I can see in the distance fresh daffodil buds emerging through the rain sodden soil. A sign of new life which gladdens my heart. The church clock chimes ten times which is useful as I appear to have left my watch at home.

A strange dog jumps out of nowhere. A lively spaniel who seems to have escaped from its owner. The spaniel wants to make friends with George, but George shows complete disinterest. George prefers cats, and the over excited spaniel looks nothing like a cat. I can see Spaniel's human owner running breathlessly up the path, shouting a strange name that neither I or the spaniel can understand, and I wonder why the spaniel keeps running away. Does he hate his weird sounding name? Within a few minutes the pair are reunited and George and I are left alone again, glad of the return of the peace and quiet. George is particularly happy to be free of the spaniel who sniffed his bottom within thirty seconds of meeting. There are times I'm glad I'm not a dog just for that reason.

***

The wind picks up ferociously as I continue my walk across the field. I turn my head into the breeze as it swirls around me and I wonder if Mum is here. Momentarily I feel her presence and breathe in the cool Yorkshire air. A tiny leaf settles in my hair and I decide to leave it there, just in case it's a present from Mum. I wonder if grief can send you crazy? Do I really think

Mum popped a leaf in my hair? I guess it doesn't matter if she did or not. What matters is that I feel comforted. I continue my walk with the leaf trapped in my hair, resolving to leave it there as long as I can. On arriving home I look in the mirror to discover the leaf has gone. Perhaps it wasn't a gift from Mum. Perhaps it was just a fragile leaf caught on the wind. I feel disappointed and bereft. I wanted it to be a sign from Mum, a sign that she is still here with me. Never mind, there will be more leaves.

The kettle boils for my morning cup of tea and I watch it closely. What a fantastic invention. So much easier than watching a pan of water on the oven hob, waiting for the bubbles to rise, which indicate that our cup of tea is not far away. I read that it costs a lot of money to boil a kettle. I must remember not to overfill it.

***

The wilting daffodils on the dining table continue their journey into daffodil heaven. I wonder if I can do anything to save them. I give them fresh water but an hour later they look worse than ever. I want to blame the water, but I know in my heart their time on earth is at an end. My heart sinks knowing I am helpless in my quest to revive them. I think of Mum and how I thought wishful thinking would save her too. My wishful thinking was not enough. Sometimes we have to accept the inevitable, I guess. I say goodnight and thank you to them before heading up to bed, knowing I will have yet another funeral to attend to in the morning.

***

Three things I am grateful for today.

1 Daffodils that brighten springtime.

2 Sympathy cards that show us how much we are loved.

3 My life with Mum.

Chapter Three

Friday 24th March 2023

The start of the weekend and I'm celebrating in style with a trip to the dentist, following a few days of toothache. An imminent family holiday to Switzerland means I need to get it checked before I travel. It's exactly a week since the funeral, and quite honestly, the last place I want to be is at the dentist. However, toothache has no respect for a person's state of mind, and so I find myself in the car, on a reluctant visit to the dentist to have the toothache assessed. As I drive I think about how the world keeps turning, regardless of loss and grief. Shops still open, trains still run, children go to school and toothache still visits us when we least expect it. When our calm world is hit by uncontrollable grief, we half expect everything to stop, to pause, while we catch our breath and gather our thoughts. We watch as the world continues to run as normal, while we cry alone, wishing our loved one would come back to us. Toothache is perhaps the most disrespectful of all. Annoying, intrusive and painful. I hate toothache, even more than I have ever hated it, coming into my life as an unwelcome visitor while my tears still lie wet on my cheeks. But, here we are. Like it or not.

***

Parking the car, I walk to the pay machine for my ticket. A man with a furrowed brow is fumbling with the machine and swearing under his breath.

'Godamn council, always charging us a fortune for parking. Bloody robbers.'

He grabs his ticket, but drops his money in the process. I watch various coins roll down the hill. He gives chase, almost falling over his untied shoelace shouting, 'bloody Council!' I'm not sure the Council are bothered what 'Mr Untied Shoelace Man' thinks of car parking charges, but they are probably very happy that he has just contributed to their annual Christmas party.

***

In the dentist waiting room there is a diminutive woman tapping her feet nervously while chewing her lip. I feel sorry for her, however I can't really comfort her as I too am crumbling inside at the thought of the next thirty minutes. I watch the tropical fish swimming around their tank surrounded by exotic plants, and I imagine myself swimming in warm Caribbean waters. One fish looks like Nemo from the Disney film and I half expect him to start talking. He remains silent. However, I do hear the dental assistant call my name and I say goodbye to Nemo who completely ignores my current angst.

As I sit in the dreaded dentist's chair I wonder what Nemo is doing right now. My attention is taken by the thoughtfully placed tv screen on the ceiling, supposedly to help calm patients down as they lie in the chair. It doesn't work for me. I prefer to think of Nemo floating in his warm, tropical world, enjoying the tranquility of his cosy tank, eating delicious fish food. Sometimes we only need the simplest of things in life to keep us happy and fulfilled. As the dentist starts up the drill, I concentrate hard and think of warm turquoise water and tropical fish swimming gracefully without a care in the world. A loud, grating noise interrupts my mindful thoughts. The visualisation doesn't work effectively, but the drill does.

***

Walking back to the car an hour later I see a teenage girl arguing with her Mother. The situation seems to be escalating the closer I get.

'No Saffron, you CANNOT stay out till 11 o'clock tonight!'

The teenage girl with long blond hair stamps her feet and flushes from the neck up.

'But Mother, I am not a child anymore. I am sixteen. I demand to be treated like an adult.'

Whispers follow as the mother tries to calm the girl and reason with her. As I pass the stressed out duo I hear Saffron say,

Ok, Mother. Ten o clock then. But can I borrow fifty quid please?'

I come to the quick conclusion that perhaps Saffron is not quite ready to be an adult yet and still regards her parents as her own personal bank.

***

Stuck in a traffic jam I observe a woman dressed in a crimson red coat stood on the pavement, looking at her mobile phone. She looks sad and tearful and I wonder if she has just received bad news, or maybe she is reminiscing about good times. I do that a lot since Mum died. I look at old photos, supposedly to make me feel better. It doesn't work. I usually end up crying. The woman in the red coat glances up at the sky deep in thought. I wonder if she is looking for inspiration, or maybe she is looking for a loved one who has passed away. I do that too. I haven't seen anyone yet.

***

On the other side of the road I see two men dressed in paint splattered clothing, holding fish and chips, wrapped in paper. They are obviously hungry as they dip their hands into their precious packages, greedily devouring the battered chips. They eat in silence, but in harmony, and now I have a craving for fish and chips, which I know won't go away until I have some.

***

In the fish shop, three miles down the road I patiently queue for my supper, although there are six people in front of me, which makes me panic slightly that they might run out of fish. The server looks tired and weary as she packs fish and chips like a robot, hardly stopping to breathe, until she gently scoops the mushy peas into a polystyrene tub which seems to relax her. Perhaps she likes the colour green. I reach the front of the queue and as I start to talk I realise I can't actually move my mouth properly. Damn dentist. I forgot. No fish and chips for me tonight. I drive home slowly, feeling despondent, hoping I have some soup in the fridge for later.

***

As I draw the curtains in my bedroom I become aware of the sweet noise of an owl as it sings its night time song. His 'twit twoo' echoes penetrating the cool March air. I imagine he is talking directly to me, reassuring me that everything will be ok. I tell him that he needs to work harder, as right now I feel lost and bewildered. I yawn widely and curse the dentist yet again. Tomorrow is a new day.

***

Three things I am grateful for today.

1 Dentists who help keep our teeth healthy.

2 Fish and chips which are perhaps the most comforting food on the planet.

3 The song of the owl, comforting me as I fall asleep.

Chapter Four

Monday 27th March 2023

Preparing for our holiday has been difficult, which is not surprising given my circumstances over the last few weeks. My usual packing routine is disturbed by strange, guilty thoughts of leaving Mum behind, while I travel eight hundred miles through Europe to Switzerland. I understand I'm not leaving her as she has already gone, but still my mind feels unable to accept this, and so, the constant torment continues. I am glad of my daily routine of journalling as it gives me a quiet space to record my thoughts and observations. It gently ushers me into a more mindful way of life, to take notice of the little things, to really appreciate everything.

As I pack my case, my weary mind returns to holiday memories of many years ago. It all seemed so simple then, the packing I mean. I glance down at my holdall that contains all the electrical equipment I need for a month in Switzerland. My laptop, headphones, Ipad, plug adaptors and of course all the chargers and other gizmos that go with it all. I love the technology that makes our life so much easier, but sometimes it feels like a burden weighing down an already heavy life. Still, we must embrace advancements in order to keep up with the complexities of the modern world. I sigh. So why doesn't it feel like it's the right thing to do? The constant angst of preparing for my holiday is relieved slightly by the fact that we have an overnight stop in the UK before we catch the Eurotunnel to mainland Europe. This prepares me for a slow exit, away from Mum, although every mile travelled away from home feels difficult and makes me feel anxious.

Watching the world go by as we travel quickly on the motorway, I am lulled into a dreamy state by the rhythmic appearance of a multitude of patchwork green fields as they flash by in a blur. I wonder if I am being watched as we travel. Perhaps a lone rabbit is hiding in the hedge by the side of the road. Is he waiting for a break in the traffic so he can cross the road to the other side? I hope he stays where he is. Dear Mr Rabbit, the grass is not always greener!

We stop three hours later at a motorway services area. A visit to the Ladies and the coffee shop soon restores my flagging spirits. Sipping my decaffeinated latte at a worn and unstable wooden table, I glance round at my fellow travellers, in my quest to keep trying to reconnect with the world I lost a few weeks ago. I am aware that my surroundings seem unreal, unsure of how everything fits together. Listening to everyday conversations, mundane and otherwise, helps relieve the confusion of my tired and grieving mind. I smile inwardly, aware that my fellow travellers in this coffee shop know nothing of my torment, or conversely, just how much they are helping me distract myself from the dark abyss of loss. I quietly say 'thank you' to them, as they go about their life, here in this motorway coffee shop.

***

On the next table to me, a young mother looks to to the sky, maybe for divine intervention, maybe for a little inspiration. Her young daughter, aged about three, sips warm milk from a small paper cup, smiling broadly as the milk creates froth round her mouth. The mother laughs, gently wiping the excess milk with a white napkin. The young girl grimaces. The mother persists.

'Molly, don't be silly. I need to clean you up.'

Molly pulls away, frowning and then proceeds to take another long, noisy slurp from her cup, creating yet another frothy mess on her face. The mother sighs, dropping the napkin on the table.

'I give up.' she whispers under her breath, raising her eyes upwards once more.

***

An elderly couple huddle closely together on the next table, concentrating on their milky lattes. The woman winks and suddenly produces a small plastic bag from which she brings out two custard cream biscuits. She passes one of the biscuits to her male companion who pauses, then looks round surreptitiously, making sure the coffee shop staff can't see his sweet treat. The two giggle to each other, excited that they have managed to sneak in food to the coffee shop when there is a stark, prominent sign above them saying 'Please do not consume your own food.' I feel happy for them that they are breaking the rules. At their age I think this is momentous and definitely worth doing. My Mum often broke rules as she got older. She had a carefree, 'couldn't care less' attitude and I know she would be cheering on the Custard Cream couple for their illicit behaviour.

The staff are too busy to notice the older couple secretly eating their custard cream biscuits. In fact, I'm not sure they would care even if they knew. A young brunette girl is stood behind the till taking orders from weary travellers, who are desperate for a coffee fix after their long journey. She looks sad and apathetic as she takes constant, consecutive orders of lattes, cappuccinos and americanos with hot milk. Her badge reveals her name is Joy, but from where I'm sat, I can't see any joy in her life right now. Joy uses the till with such swift efficiency that I think she has been doing this job for longer than she can remember. Boredom is written across the pretty, young face, and I just hope that Joy can find the will and determination to leave the job of doom, and find something else that makes her heart sing. Something tells me it certainly isn't taking coffee orders on a busy Monday afternoon on the M1.

***

Arriving at our first hotel for the night, I drop wearily onto the comfortable bed, with its deep mattress and soft pillows that hug my head and shoulders. I lay staring at the ceiling, already feeling tired of travelling, sighing deeply, knowing there is still a long way to go. The kettle boils quickly and soon I am clutching a hot cup of tea, the steam warming my cold face. My Mum always used to say that a cup of tea solves everything, and slowly I am beginning to understand what she meant. Sipping on a cup of tea gives us time to stand back from life, from problems, from difficulties and issues that need resolving. A cup of tea is universal. Whatever our situation is, we can all enjoy a cup of comforting tea together. My eyes fill with warm water, emotions now overwhelming me. I wish Mum were here. I lay back on the bed and invite a peaceful sleep to wash over me.

***

Three things I am grateful for today.

1 The ability to travel freely.

2 Technology that connects us with others.

3 Hot tea.

Chapter Five

Tuesday 28th March 2023

Holidays usually begin with early morning starts, high stress levels and half consumed cups of tea. It is no different for me, as we leave the comfort of our Folkestone hotel for the Eurotunnel, which will take us across the English Channel (under it, if you want to be accurate) and onwards to our next stop in France and then Switzerland. Our first check in is at the Pet Passport Centre, where we will receive confirmation that we can take our dog George with us on our European travels. The Pet Passport Centre is by far the easiest and most interesting part of the process. A multitude of dogs, cats and even ferrets queue in an orderly fashion, waiting to be checked and verified before they can set their feet (paws) in Northern France.

***

A chocolate brown labrador waits patiently in front of us, looking nonchalant about his current situation. That is, until he spots a rather interesting looking labradoodle who struts through the entrance door with an aristocratic air of superiority. Obviously the labrador believes he is the king of the Pet Passport Centre, and asserts his dominance by uncurling his neck, rather like a giraffe. The deposed labradoodle responds in the only way he can and pees rather gracefully on a sign saying 'Queue This Way.' The mortified owner quickly wipes the offending yellow evidence and glares at her dog. The queue suddenly moves and the labrador is now busy having his neck scanned, wagging his tail violently in anticipation of the treat that comes after he is successfully cleared to travel. The labradoodle is suddenly subdued and I am betting that the owner has withdrawn any treats following his indescretion. I look down at George, my own dog, silently begging him not to pee until we get outside. George waits. George is a good boy.

***

Waiting to board our train, we sit in the departure lounge. It's nothing too fancy, but has all we need before we travel, coffee, cake and rather swish toilets and not forgetting the duty free, where I get a free spray of perfume and buy a rather oversized white chocolate Toblerone.

***

A couple are sitting on the table next to us drinking a Starbucks coffee. They look tired already and they haven't even started their journey. They are both silent, glancing at the departures board every now and then. The man reaches into a Tesco carrier bag and pulls out a Kit Kat, breaking it in two and hands half to his travelling companion. She frowns.

'Isn't it rather early for chocolate?'

She reaches for his outstretched hand and takes half of the Kit Kat and pops it on the table. The man starts to eat his chocolate, slurping coffee, smiling as he does so. He watches her intently with a 'knowing' look. It isn't long before she takes her own chocolate and eats it hungrily. She sits back, content, smiling.

'Anyway, we are nearly in France and they are an hour ahead, so it's perfectly okay to have chocolate at this time in the morning.' she says sweetly.

I look at my watch. It is 7am UK time, so I know it is still only 8am in France, and I am pretty sure the French don't eat Nestle Kit Kat for breakfast, even with coffee.

***

We finally sit in our car, secure on one of the many carriages that make up the Eurotunnel train. This is the part where we put our head back and get thirty minutes nap time, while we speed onward to Calais. I unbuckle my seat belt and snuggle down in my seat, ready for departure, noticing my husband has already closed his eyes.

***

I delay closing my eyes as I am fascinated by the couple parked in front of us who have opened their boot and have started to unload various bags. The woman who is dressed casually with a windswept hairstyle, whips out a blue checked tablecover, like a magician pulling a rabbit out of a hat. Placing the cover neatly in the boot, her male companion proceeds to empty a rather stylish looking picnic basket. I am awestruck by what follows. Chintz plates and cups, floral serviettes and a selection of croissants, cheese and ham are delicately placed on the table cover. Within a couple of minutes the elegant duo are feasting on a spread fit for a king, smiling and chatting happily to each other.

I am suddenly very hungry and look longingly at them, hoping for an invite to their Eurotunnel picnic. No such invite arrives and so I reach into my bag to retrieve an angry looking, over ripe banana. I eat it while watching them consume the last of the delicious looking croissants, hoping they feel guilty at my pathetic breakfast. Of course, they don't feel guilty, but I make a mental note to get more organised next time. I wonder what Mr and Mrs KitKat would think of this picnic arrangement. Maybe they wouldn't? Maybe they enjoy a KitKat breakfast every time they travel? The light streams into the carriage as we reach France, and I watch Mr and Mrs Perfect Picnic pack away the remnants of their breakfast. They smile at me as they shake the tablecover free of croissant crumbs. I return the smile, but secretly I am annoyed at myself that I didn't think of a delicious Eurotunnel picnic for us. I nudge my husband to wake up ready for disembarkment.

'Did I miss anything' he asks sleepily.

'Only croissants dear.'

***

Three things I am grateful for today.

1 Pets are allowed to travel abroad with us.

2 Eurotunnel, so I don't have to go on a plane (I hate flying.)

3 Being inspired by other people's lives.

Chapter Six

Wednesday 29th March 2023

Crisp fresh air, snow topped mountains, pine scented forests can only mean one thing. Switzerland. As a regular visitor here, I never tire of its beauty and peaceful environment. My wish for this holiday is to recharge, refresh and heal from the deep trauma of the last three months. I am hopeful that this will happen, but sadness has already set in to my tired body. I am always in awe of the power of nature and looking at the mountains from my Swiss balcony, I am suddenly overcome with intense grief. My whole body aches, my heart literally hurts as I long to see my beloved Mother again. The beauty of my view triggers emotions that I have been holding in for weeks. The reality of the situation consumes me and I crumple in a heap and sob heavily.

Sometime later, I hold a cup of Swiss hot chocolate in my hand, gently inhaling the comforting aroma of my favourite drink. I look again at the majestic Alps towering over the landscape, the tiny Swiss villages and I breathe deeply in reverance to the all mighty and powerful landscape. I feel my fragility, my smallness and yet, I imagine I am being held by the mountains, protected in some way from the ferocity of grief.

The sunset creeps up slowly and I watch the most wonderful light show created not by man, but by Mother Nature. Yellow turns to orange and then to gold, as shadows dance across the sky, heralding the arrival of evening. Peace settles across the valley and I watch as lights twinkle in tiny houses, ready for the inevitable darkness. I imagine cosy homes with local families gathering for a typical Swiss Apero and cheese fondue, punctuated by laughter and the sharing of stories after a fulfilling day. But then I realise that grief travels far and wide, and no one can escape the deep sadness of bereavement, and I pray silently for all those Swiss people who may be grieving tonight, much like myself. I suddenly remember the saying, 'after the darkness comes the light' and so, clutching the remains of my hot chocolate, I head to bed for an early night, ready for a new start tomorrow. I know this grief will still be with me, but I remain positive that tomorrow, the sadness will sleep for a little while, allowing me to see the glimmers of light that I need so badly.

***

Three things I am grateful for today.

1 Switzerland, the most beautiful country in the world.

2 Swiss Caotina hot chocolate.

3 Sharing my grief with others, regardless of age, background or nationality. We all grieve.

Chapter Seven

Thursday 30th March 2023

Following a restless night, I watch the sunrise as it creeps slowly over the mountains, peeking out, hesitant about the new day, much like myself at the moment. After a difficult, emotional day yesterday, I am determined to fight this life sapping melancholy, and resume my mindful observations of life around me. My journal is my friend, my therapist, and so my notebook snuggles in my pocket and together we continue our journey. I leave the chalet after breakfast, grateful for the feeling of warmth on my face, eager to find any pockets of joy in this new day.

***

I see a herd of cows ambling lazily in a newly cut meadow, the smell of fresh cut grass tickles my nose. I am fascinated by the sight and sound of huge bells that swing from the necks of every Swiss cow. The cows walk together and in harmony, in peace and without stress, much like the philosophy of the Swiss nation who are recognised for their calmness and neutrality. The bells are poetic in their ringing and I find them calming to my frazzled mind. I am unsure why, but the sound makes me smile and lifts my spirits.

***

A man dressed in work overalls sits on a sunny terrace drinking from a large pot cup that looks as though it has seen better days. He is talking in Swiss German to a black and white cat that is sat by his side. The cat warmly acknowledges the man by soft meowing and rubbing his body across the man's legs. The man laughs and pats the cat's head gently. They are enjoying each others company, with a natural affection for each other. I stop to wonder why human relationships can't be that simple? I walk away smiling to myself, leaving the two of them alone in their friendship.

***

In the distance, paragliders swirl and twirl in the air, performing the foxtrot with the ominously looming mountains close by. Transfixed, I marvel at their bravery and aerial finesse as they glide through the cold Swiss air. I wonder if fear is uppermost in their mind as they skillfully negotiate their descent? Or do they manage to use their fearful emotions to their advantage, so that they feel empowered and invincible? They fly with incredible grace and poise, descending with such ease, and there is a moment when they appear to morph into a giant bird. I wonder if the local birdlife watch them with awe or even humour, at their attempts to soar through the clouds. As the human birds gather momentum as they return to the earth, I think of my own fears, those that hold me back in life or stop me in my tracks. Many humans, yes, that includes me, would never dream of paragliding, or any other extreme sport for fear of something going wrong. I guess we can all find happiness in different things, whether it is stroking a cat's head or jumping off an Alpine mountain with just a parachute to steer you to safety. Personally, I would prefer to sit with a cat on my knee. It feels safer.

***

As I walk back to my chalet I notice the man dressed in work overalls is still on his balcony, but now he has no cup in his hand. I notice the black and white cat curled up on his knee, sleeping peacefully. Both human and animal in perfect harmony. No need for extreme sports or fear driven activities. Genuine happiness can really be found in the simplest of things. And now for my own slice of happiness. A piece of Swiss strawberry tart washed down with a hot chocolate, of course. It's the little things.

***

It is 2am. Sleep evades me. My thoughts are with Mum. The night is cold, so I wrap up warm and sit outside on the balcony. Looking up I am covered in a blanket of shimmering stars that glisten in the deep blue sky. I pause to make sure I breathe it all in. The stars are so close I can almost touch them, gather them in my hand and pull them close to my heart, healing the gaping hole left by my Mother's passing. The moon watches over the millions of stars like a protective mother guiding her offspring, and I too feel the warmth of her caring light. A shooting star takes me by surprise, as it breaks formation from its fellow stars, much like a fledgling fleeing from the nest. The tops of the snowy mountains are lit by the moon and her rays, like a floodlight on the stage of a West End play, but here the star of the show is the Jungfrau, one of the highest mountains in Switzerland.

I feel privileged watching this special performance of the night sky in all her beauty. While most people sleep, I am enjoying the most fantastic spectacle that nature can produce. We often hear the phrase 'nature heals' without actually thinking too deeply about it, or how it works. Tonight has proven that there is no blueprint, no detailed plan, no intricate instructions. Just nature doing what it does best. Offering hope and comfort to those who need it.

Thank you Mother Nature for tonight. Thank you for helping me heal.

***

Three things I am grateful for today.

1 Swiss cows and their tuneful bells.

2 Witnessing the profound relationship between human and animal.

3 Swiss mountains, especially the Jungfrau.

Chapter Eight

Wednesday 5th April 2023

After a week in Switzerland, I am still feeling profoundly unsettled and I am struggling to sleep. Homesickness has kicked in as I find myself craving for home, family and familiarity. I find myself looking at photographs of my daughters and their family and I am longing to see them. I miss heartfelt hugs from my grandchildren and the thought of not being able to see them all right now fills my eyes with tears. My heart is actually hurting at the distance between us and I cry frequently at the thought of it. I conclude that it has been a mistake to come away on holiday so soon after the funeral, and so, we have decided to return home early. We will leave in a few days after the Easter weekend. In the meantime I focus on my writing and seek out interesting subjects to add to my journal.

Coffee shops are always a fantastic base for writing inspiration. A cup of milky coffee complimented with delicious cake and a prominent seat, is all I need to observe real life characters and their daily routine. I smile thinking of all the people I have observed over the years, who have inspired me to write and helped me create an interesting piece of writing. Oh, how I wish I could thank every person who had unknowingly helped my creative process. If you are one of my 'subjects' and are reading this book, I thank you.

I am now firmly positioned at an outside table at a wonderful coffee shop in Interlaken. My steaming milky coffee sits on the linen covered table before me, alongside the most delicious piece of chocolate cake. It looks like I will be here for some time. Refills on the ready.

***

An elegant woman of about sixty years sits on the next table, dressed in a long, black wool coat and puffing on a cigarette. With her red felt fedora perched on her newly coiffured hair, she reminds me of a Hollywood star of the Golden Era. She is pensive and reflective, and seems unaware of life going on around her. I'm not sure if she is sad or happy. She has a 'hard to read' face that lacks any clue as to her current mood. Suddenly, Miss Red Felt Hat catches sight of something that interests her. Her face suddenly transforms into one of spontaneous emotion, happiness and even joy. As yet, I cannot see the focus of her attention as my view is obscured by the sun umbrella at my table. I imagine a tall, distinguised gentleman, her lover perhaps? A secret assignation of two lovers shrouded in mystery and intrigue. How exciting!

A shadow appears in my eyeline, and I see the object of her attention as she recites her companion's name with excitement. My heart sinks, but leaps at the same time. There is no mysterious lover, no secret affair, not even a faithful husband. Even better, Miss Red Felt Hat has a very important date with a petite, and equally elegant woman – her mother. Their greeting to each other fills my heart with joy. They embrace and hug with such warmth, that I feel I am intruding on this perfect reunion. I lower my head for a moment, but still can't resist a peek at this adorable couple. Miss Red Felt Hat catches my eye and smiles. We may originate from different countries, but I think we both understand the powerful bond between a mother and daughter. I return to my luke-warm coffee, tuck into my cake and leave them to their joyous reunion.

***

A young boy of about ten rides his scooter in the market square, a little over-enthusiastically. His mother berates him, following a near collision with a tall, bearded man, who is thankfully nimble enough to avoid harm. The young scooter rider carries on his wilful riding, oblivious to his mother's concerns. Dodging pedestrians and waiters carrying hot coffee and cake, his anxious mother finally decides to call a halt to his antics. She grabs the scooter from his control and the young boy falls in a heap on the floor, his bereft face telling the full story of his emotions. His mother remains steadfast and tightens her grip on the offending scooter. The boy cries and stamps his feet shouting at his mother in a language I do not understand, but to be honest, I still get the gist of it. I watch the mother as she transforms into a strong-willed, 'never to be beaten' woman.

I admire her determination and natural ability to handle her son with such grace and ease. After a few minutes the young boy accepts his fate and approaches his mother with tears in his eyes. A gentle and quiet conversation ensues, followed by warm hugs and smiles. However, the mother still keeps the scooter in her grasp, as the boy sits quietly drinking a glass of warm milk. I smile, recognising that most mothers have this special and extraordinary ability to diffuse a difficult situation, quickly and peacefully.

***

Ordering a milky hot chocolate, I watch the marketplace drift into a snooze as people empty their coffee cups and make their way home. People with such different lives, like ants scurrying back to the place they came from, familiar and comforting, a place to cast off the worries of the day, like old shoes that no longer have purpose. I think of all the stories that each person could tell – tales of happiness, disappointment, joy and grief. We can never escape different emotions over the course of our life, but we must learn how to manage them, like the young boy with the scooter. I make a mental note of this to help me through my own journey of grief. I must learn how to manage it.

***

My next thought is rather more wayward. I really want to get a scooter when I get home as it looks like so much fun. As I head back to the chalet I decide I will check out adult scooters on the internet, but promise myself I would be slightly more responsible riding one than the young Swiss boy. The image of me riding a scooter in Yorkshire at the age of sixty fills my heart with joy and dread at the same time. I wonder if there are scooter lessons for women my age? My dream of becoming a 'scooter chick' is somewhat dampened on arriving back at the chalet when the internet informs me that riding a scooter is illegal in the UK, unless on private land. To be honest I'm not sure it would be safe riding on UK roads anyway, with the presence of so many potholes. It would certainly have been fun though!

I collapse into my cosy bed, warmed by the presence of my hot water bottle and I think of slow coffee dates, speeding scooters and my mother dressed in a red felt fedora. It has been an interesting day and I wish Mum could have been here with me to experience it all. My heart sinks, as it does most days lately, with the realisation that Mum is not coming back. Like the young boy on the scooter, I have to accept certain facts of life as the truth, even though it makes me sad. And yet, tonight, I still despise the fact that we have to say goodbye to loved ones, permanently. I remember someone saying to me at my Mum's funeral, 'Oh, she had a good life and lived to an old age.' Yes, I was blessed to have her here for so long, but the loss is still felt the same. Death is so final, and yet my heart is having trouble believing that tonight. Still, there is always tomorrow.

***

Three things I am grateful for today.

1 Swiss coffee shops.

2 My three daughters who make me proud every single day.

3 The love between a mother and daughter.

Chapter Nine

Thursday 13th April 2023

I arrive home in the UK after an uneventful return trip from Switzerland to be greeted by reduced Easter eggs and a recording of Easter Parade, starring Judy Garland. My mother loved this film and I settle down on the sofa to watch it, accompanied by a Dairy Milk Easter egg that was only £1.50. Two hours later with a full and rather sickly stomach, I take the dog out for a walk singing Easter Parade at the top of my voice, promising myself that I NEVER want to see or eat chocolate ever again. I know this is a lie but I say it anyway.

The air feels clear, but my thoughts return to Switzerland, already missing the brisk fresh air of the Alps. I try to walk quickly, but my dog George has other ideas and we both drift into a slow, rhythmic walk. As George leads the way, happily wagging his tail, I am reminded how much humans differ from animals. George and my Mum were great friends and I know he was a great comfort to her. I wonder if he realises she is no longer here, or is his memory unable to hold onto feelings of loss? It's a mystery and probably always will be, but his obvious happiness walking down the road, a few miles from home, makes me feel lucky and blessed to have him in my life, especially now.

***

A man with a heavily tattooed right arm is painting his front door with a rather small paint brush. He tilts his head from side to side, trying to get a better look at the door, often standing back to admire his art work. I love his confidence, but someone needs to tell him that it is a wooden door and not the Sistine Chapel. Also, more importantly, someone also needs to inform him that he has used two different shades of blue, and it currently looks like a stick of rock. I certainly don't think Michelangelo has anything to worry about.

***

As I approach a bus stop I hear a loud noise behind me. It is a double decker red bus. The bus doors are flung open and the driver dressed in all blue shouts at me.

'Hurry up love, if you're getting on.'

I politely inform him that I don't want the bus.

'So why are you waiting at the bus stop then?'

I try to explain that I am, in fact, merely walking past the bus stop and not 'waiting.' The bus driver grunts some inexplicable words and I realise this conversation is going nowhere, and so, I smile sweetly apologising for 'hovering' at the bus stop. The bus driver sighs so loudly he sinks down in his seat and actually loses two inches in height. The doors close and he drives off, rolling his eyes as he does so. I decide from now on I will change my morning dog walk to avoid all bus stops and so as not to mislead the bus driver. I may even study the bus timetable to make sure I avoid the aforementioned bus. I've never avoided a bus before, so this could be a whole new experience.

***

Next to the bus stop a tall, lanky girl dressed in all black sits on a wooden bench, engrossed in a serious sounding telephone conversation. The Goth like figure looks pasty white as though she has just seen a ghost. I rebuke myself, remembering that this is exactly the look she is going for. If she wasn't engaged on the telephone, I would probably tell her that she looks lovely, just to cheer her up. From the way the conversation is going, I think she may need cheering up very soon.

'Bram, I cannot believe that you have lost your teeth! I only bought them last week. Have you looked in the junk drawer in the kitchen?'

Miss Goth lapses into silence and I can only imagine Bram is explaining the demise of the lost teeth. Miss Goth, obviously used to the hapless Bram sighs loudly, dropping her shoulders violently.

'How can you ever be the coolest Dracula in Whitby if you keep losing your teeth!?'

The call ends abruptly and I conclude that I have led a very sheltered life, but I make a mental note to visit Whitby again very soon.

***

George makes friends with a chalky white and brown Cocker Spaniel in the park. His new friend is called Cup. I am drawn into conversation with Cup's owner, even though I am desperate for some peace and quiet time. Owning a dog always brings the opportunity to converse with other dog owners, usually when you least want it. However, I am polite and I make small talk about the weather, the state of the potholes on the local roads and the price of bananas. Feeling terribly British,

I try steer the topic to Cup and his unusual name. It always amazes me how many quirky dog names there are nowadays.

'Cup? Aye. It's a great name isn't it? A strong British name, reflecting strong country breeding.'

I smile weakly, looking down at Cup who is currently trying to hump George, with no care in the world that George happens to be a male castrated dog.

'Hey Cup, stop that! What's wrong with ya lad? Are ye gay?'

Cup stares at his owner with that knowing look in his eye – 'Look mate, it's 2023 and I can be whatever I want to be.'

Sad to disturb this treasured owner and dog moment, I ask the question once again.

'So why is he called Cup?'

Puffing out his chest, the owner of Cup announces with great pride.

'Oh, his sister was called Cake, but she's no longer with us.'

Offering my apologies and condolences for the loss of Cake, I am abruptly stopped in my tracks by Cup's owner.

'Oh no love. Don't worry. Cake is alive and well. She's now living with my ex–wife down south. When we got divorced we split everything in half, including the dogs.'

I sigh, ever grateful that they had two dogs to split in half, rather than just one. I smile broadly at Cup, just to let him know that however much he hates his name, it could have been a lot worse!

***

I arrive home to read a difficult email from the local council about an unpaid bill from Mum's estate. I ignore it, not wanting to remind myself of the empty chair or my empty heart. I have learnt over the past few months that organisations can be ruthless when dealing with the bereaved and heartbroken. Whatever happened to compassion and care for a fellow human being who is in the midst of grieving? I return to my computer and delete the email that is giving me great angst. They know where I live. They can write to me.

***

Three things I am grateful for today.

1 Easter eggs

2 Old Hollywood films.

3 The ability to delete an email when it suits me.

Chapter Ten

Sunday 16th April 2023

It has been a difficult week. Having to deal with 'sadmin' of a loved one is traumatic in itself as we try and get to grips with a loved one's finances, house contents, unpaid bills, and any other meaningless activites that constantly remind us that they have gone. Not gone for a day or a week, but forever. Grief is a rollercoaster playing tricks with your mind and fragility. It weaves its way into your emotions and then strikes like a sharpened pencil into your heart, twisting and digging deep, until you can't take any more. But we have to carry on. Society says so.

I wonder if we could revert to the old way of mourning, when the recently bereaved would wear black outfits giving a signal to the world, 'I am grieving. Be gentle with me as I navigate my way through this muddle.' Sadly, there is no period of mourning, no donning of black outfits and we are expected to pull ourselves together once the funeral has been held. Today I am going out for the day, to get lost in the Yorkshire Dales, not literally lost, but lost enough to escape from the crowds and my innermost thoughts.

It is Sunday and in the distance I can hear church bells signalling the start of the regular church service. This great British tradition is still upheld in many corners of the UK, but is especially so in the North of England where bell ringing is still maintained by generations of the same family. In my own village, I often walk to the churchyard to listen to bell ringing practice night which is held every Thursday. I am enchanted by the dulcit tones of the old bells and I often imagine a small group of people stood in a cold Norman bell tower guiding the heavy bell ropes, praying that they don't pull the ropes at the wrong time. I often dream of becoming a bell ringer myself, but the stress of getting it right would be too overwhelming. It's not exactly easy to cover it up if you get it wrong. I also have visions of being swept upwards by the strong ropes and hanging from the bell tower like the Hunchback of Notre Dame. I also recently watched a film where members of a church bell ringing group were killed one by one, by a crazy psychopath. Maybe it's easier to keep out of the bell tower. It seems the less traumatic path.

We arrive just before lunchtime in a small Yorkshire village. Traditional stone walls weave their way gently round the village centre, proudly asserting their claim of belonging to the group of the strongest walls in history. I'm not sure the Romans would agree, but I love the Yorkshire confidence. The large village is awash with cosy tea rooms, and so it is not long before we are settled, eager for a delicious lunch and a nice warm drink.

***

A rather robust couple on the next table are dressed head to toe in trendy hiking gear and reading Ordnance Survey maps. They talk quietly, but every few minutes I catch a few choice words.

'Oh Nigel. That looks an awful long way. What if I need the toilet? You know how my bladder is. I just have to pee every so often. I can't help it.'

I see Nigel rolling his eyes. Nigel has obviously been through this scenario before. He has that look of resignation. I personally don't think Nigel is very supportive of his partner's bladder issue and this disturbs me. I remind myself that when I am absorbed in observational journalling, I must not get too involved in the lives of others. This is an issue I find difficult to accept and today is no exception.

I must admit I am slowly losing my appetite for the tuna salad I have just ordered, with visions of this poor woman running to relieve herself, while hiking in the Yorkshire Dales. Twenty minutes later the couple grab their over sized rucksacks and head out into the warm sunshine. I watch them walk down the high street together, still conversing excitedly, probably about the woman's weak bladder. She is waving her arms violently like a helicopter, while Nigel strides purposefully like a man possessed. Personally if I were her, I would dump Nigel at the nearest kissing gate and find myself a nice cosy hotel, enjoy a hot bath and a good book, and most importantly a luxurious en suite bathroom, so she need never fear about getting caught short again!

***

An hour later as we are strolling round the Yorkshire Dales, I think of the 'Bladder Couple'. I wonder what their life is like back home, what job do they do and what family do they have? During my time observing and journalling I am always conscious that what I see is only a tiny glimpse of a person's life. I feel honoured to be part of their life, but also aware that each one of them might, at any time, be suffering grief and loss, just like me. Often we don't share these most intimate emotions with others. We pretend we are strong and resourceful, and we carry on with our fixed smiles and positive attitude, while inside many of us are broken, hanging on by a thread. Grief is so private, so personal and so raw. How sad that we often feel unable to share this important period of life.

As I retire to my bedroom worn out by the long hike, I am suddenly grateful for my own situation, my cosy bed, my soft cotton sheets and my warm bathroom. As I visit my own bathroom, I think of Nigel's companion, hoping she was ok today and hoping she found a toilet when she most needed it.

***

Three things I am grateful for today.

1 Church bells.

2 My warm, cosy house and especially my bathroom.

3 The lady in the cafe, for reminding me that it's okay to have a weak bladder.

Chapter Eleven

Saturday 22nd April 2023

Today I am attending a calligraphy workshop with my dearest friend, Sandie. I am most excited by this as I love to learn anything new and creative. My friend however, is not so excited, and I know she has only come with me to support me, as I journey through my grief. In fact, Sandie has actually bought me this calligraphy workshop as a gift, as a way to help me through this difficult time. I do have the best, supportive friends!

The workshop is being held in a large luxury hotel and my first stop is the Ladies Room. Don't all ladies do this just to check out the decor, at least? I have always found the conversation in the Ladies Room inspiring to a creative like myself. Women huddled together in a private room away from the prying ears of men, always let their guard down and reveal their true authentic self. It really is a revelation and provides a deep insight into the personality of a woman. For an observational journaller like myself, the Ladies Room is the perfect place to listen and learn.

***

Blonde Lady 1: 'I've told him! I am not going to meet his ex wife. Why would I do that? Men are such idiots!'

Blonde Lady 2 : 'Maybe he wants to show you off? Show her how pretty you are!'

The two women fall silent, preferring to adjust their make up and rearrange their hair, which already looks perfect to me. As I leave the Ladies Room, I silently pray that the meeting with the ex-wife goes well, but I have my doubts.

***

The calligraphy class starts and within five minutes my friend is having a slight panic at how difficult it seems to be. I have to admit it does seem complicated, but right now I am enjoying the challenge as it takes me away from thinking about Mum. Plus, I believe creativity is good for the mind, as it gives us a feeling of self worth when we complete a creative project.

I look at my fellow calligraphy students and I can feel their enthusiasm at learning a new creative skill. They talk excitedly and I see one lady waving her calligraphy pen in the air like she is conducting an orchestra. Her friend is busy practicing the letter A on the scrap paper, whooping with delight as she successfully draws a letter that does indeed resemble the letter A. I am tempted to remind her that there are another 25 letters to go, plus numbers and it has taken her an hour to master that one letter. I think it's going to be a long afternoon.

We take a break from pens, ink and grimacing at our lack of calligraphy skills, and we all meet in a room drinking hot cups of tea and eating cream scones on delicate white china plates. Somehow, the great British tradition of eating cream scones, along with learning the art of calligraphy seems a good combination. Although a cream tea is perfect at any time of day, in my humble opinion. The ladies in the group start a conversation which I have heard so many times before, but with no obvious conclusion to the question.

'Do you put jam on first or cream?'

'Ooh, I'm not sure. What does everyone think? Shall we have a vote on it?'

'Does it matter which way you do it?'

'Yes! It really does!'

The group appear divided on the subject, emotions are triggered, and I conclude that sometimes it is best to move on from tricky conversations such as jam before cream, or visa versa, before it gets out of hand.

We return to the classroom for part two and I return to my struggles with the letter G. As we are in a rather classy hotel I refrain from swearing, but I am tempted, as my letter G looks nothing like it should do. I push back my chair to take a rest from it and then I have a wild thought that my laptop can actually write in a calligraphy font, so I may not need to learn this after all. Sometimes I love technology!

The workshop ends with lots of laughter and the realisation that calligraphy cannot be mastered in just a few hours in a hotel in deepest Yorkshire. I watch as the others sit back admiring their efforts, with some more honest than others.

'Do you think I can write 100 wedding invitations by the end of July?'

'Personally I would get a professional to do it. You don't want the added stress.'

***

I have to agree. Leave it to the professionals. As for me, I still haven't nailed the letter G and I'm not sure I ever will. As my mother always used to say 'you can't be good at everything!'

Sandie and I leave the workshop, smiling, having enjoyed a fun filled day. I am excited to try my new learned skill when I get home, but Sandie is less enthusiastic, although she hides it well, for about five minutes. As we step out of the hotel's entrance, she hands me her calligraphy pen and bottle of ink, and with the sweetest smile tells me she has no use for it. However, we both agree we have had a wonderful day, learning something new and exciting, relaxing in a fabulous hotel and filling our tummies with cream scones. Whether we go on to write calligraphy style or not, doesn't really matter. What matters is quality time spent with good friends, enjoying life and finding joy in the everyday. I am slowly learning that joy can honestly be found in the smallest things. Most of us spend our days in a haze of meetings, appointments and hurried walks. Taking life at a slower pace and viewing the world with open eyes really can help lighten our mood. Today was a good example of that. Today was a good day.

***

Three things I am grateful for today.

1 The ability to write, in fancy lettering or not.

2 Cream scones – jam first, of course.

3 Friends like Sandie, who just make my world a brighter place.

Chapter Twelve

Thursday 27th April 2023

Packing again, but this time only for an overnight stay. I often think at my age I should have this packing lark down to a fine art. The truth is, I don't. The excitement of a trip away is muted by the stress of having to determine what clothes to take, and making sure I have enough medication to last the duration of the holiday. This last point always causes angst. I'm not sure why, as today's trip is only a few miles from home, so I can always pop back if I need to.

I can hear my Mum's voice looming large in my head. 'Be prepared for every eventuality, you never know what might happen.' I frequently asked her what she meant by this and she would retell me stories of the Second World War, and how scared she was when she heard enemy aircraft overhead. However, today I can safely say that I don't think there will be any German Stukas flying over the UK tonight, so I bundle a few things in an overnight bag, rather haplessly, I might add, and I jump in the car for the short journey to the hotel.

The journey is short and uneventful and I am soon settled in one of my favourite hotels in Yorkshire. As my husband is at the hotel for a business convention, I am excited to have the evening to myself where I can wander around the hotel, eat delicious food and observe some of the guests, while looking for inspiration for my creative writing.

The hotel bar is always a great base for observing people and listening in on those important conversations (quite by accident, of course!). My chair of choice is cosy and welcoming and I snuggle down ready for the evening entertainment to start.

***

'Darling, please order me a pink gin. I'm exhausted after all that shopping.'

I congratulate myself in being at the right place at the right time. This is a wonderful start to my evening. Mrs Pink Gin is draped in a velvet armchair opposite my own chair. Dressed in a classic petal pink silk dress, she oozes glamour, and I suddenly feel rather underdressed in my Marks and Spencers floral outfit. Her companion sits resplendent in mustard linen trousers and a country style tweed jacket. I am hooked and am now emotionally invested in this picture perfect couple. I blink quickly to remind myself this is Yorkshire 2023 and not some Hollywood movie of the Golden Era.

As Mr Tweed Jacket heads for the bar, Mrs Pink Gin fingers her cream pearls rather seductively, casting her eyes slowly around the room. Her eyes stop at the sight of me, just for a second, and then she carries on her perusal of the room. I can only imagine what she thinks of little old me, unruly hair, a high street dress (from the sale rack last year) and white trainers that have seen better days.

A few minutes later, she gracefully holds the glass of gin, her long spider like fingers caressing it gently, crimson red nails providing a pop of colour. She sips the gin effortlessly as it glides down her throat like nectar to a bee. It is only then that I notice the drink matches her outfit. Is that a thing? Matching ones drink to your outfit? I glance down at my dress which is a shade of forest green, and then quickly summise that maybe I should just stick to sparkling water to be safe.

***

Tearing myself away from the glamorous couple, I watch an elderly lady in the corner of the bar retrieve a white cloth parcel from her straw bag that lies at her feet. Without breaking her concentration, she carefully unwraps the parcel to reveal a round of small, dainty sandwiches, crustless and made with white bread. She smiles at her picnic and proceeds to eat the sandwiches with careful concentration. From my chair, I deduce that her sandwich is cucumber and I applaud her in trying to keep a traditional British custom alive and kicking. I love the simplicity of her actions, her carefree attitude and her gentleness as she eats her sandwiches. I conclude that sometimes class can be found in the most unassuming of people.

***

The hotel bar is obviously a popular meeting place and it soon fills up with a variety of characters, some interesting and some not so interesting. I am feeling spoilt for choice as there is so much movement and conversations going on before me. This is when observational journalling really gets interesting. Often people and alcohol are a good mix. Inhibitions are released and the true character of a person can often surface, which is good news for a writer like myself.

***

A young woman enters the bar, looking flustered and anxious. Pacing up and down checking every chair and sofa, I am guessing that she is looking for someone. Her phone rings loudly and she answers it quickly.

'Where are you? I've been here an hour!'

'Well Tom, that's not good enough. I'm sick of coming second best to your friends. In fact, I'm going out without you.'

'No! You've lost your chance now. Stay with your stupid friends.'

Ending the call without a polite goodbye, the woman purses her lips and turns 180 degrees on her vertiginous shoes and moves to exit the bar. I am in awe of her determination to be independent. I am presuming the tight red dress she is wearing is part of the cunning plan to upset her lover. The path of true love never runs smoothly.

***

I sigh, mourning the loss of my youth, but relieved that I don't have to try squeezing into tight bodycon dresses anymore. Sometimes age can be a great leveller in life, and often it is a relief to not have the social pressures of the youth of today. However, as I look in the mirror and spot yet another wrinkle, I remember I need to buy some more expensive face cream and I sigh at the injustice of it all.

***

Three things I am grateful for today.

1 Staying in traditional British hotels.

2 Crustless cucumber sandwiches.

3 Not having to worry about fashion anymore.

Chapter Thirteen

Friday 5th May 2023

Today is the day I place Mum's ashes in my Father's grave, so they can be together. Not on my own, you understand. It all has to be done officially. A man from the Council arrives at the cemetery to make sure everything is above board and done correctly, according to the regulations. He is dressed in a slate grey suit and sombre face, clutching an A4 file with an oversized label on the front cover. I notice a long typed number on the label and wonder if it refers to my Mother. She would have hated being reduced to just a number generated by the local Council. To be honest, she didn't much care for the Council anyway. She believed that they were always up to no good, overcharging everyone with no remorse. She was probably right. I've just paid a fortune in parking fees in the local car park, just to bury my Mum today. I didn't even get a special permit.

The ceremony goes well, I guess. Just me, my husband and two of my daughters stand at the graveside, as Mr Grey Suited Council Man lowers the casket into the ground, alongside my Father's ashes. I read a poem that I wrote myself last night. I didn't even want to type it out. Somehow it seemed so final in black ink on white paper, and so I took my poem in my scrawling handwriting on a page ripped out from a journal. Mum would have preferred it in my handwriting. She loved to write free hand and she had many notebooks that contained her own poems and short stories, written with her own scrawl. My slightly haphazard approach to today would have met with her approval.

Following the brief ceremony I am reluctant to go home, and so we decide to go for lunch to a local tea room set within a garden centre. Funny place for a wake, I know, but they serve excellent quiche, which was Mum's favourite, and she particularly loved this tea room, and today is all about her.

***

A couple of elderly ladies who are sat on the next table to us are discussing the menu, grimacing and smiling simultaneously. I feel that they are having difficulty choosing their lunch and it isn't long before I am proved right.

'Doris, can we be sure the food is always freshly prepared? I do so hate those micro things. It's not natural'

'Jane, dear, I have had lunch here for the last ten years and I can spot a microwaved vegetable from a mile away. You must have faith.'

Lowered mumblings continue for the next five minutes as the two ladies keep sending the very patient waitress away, asking for more time. I am glad the running of the country is not dependent on their decision, as they discuss the menu in great detail, talking slowly, analysing every item. At last, they decide and the whole tea room visibly sighs, glad for the moment of reduced tension.

'But can you make sure that my water comes out of the tap, dear? I don't want none of this silly French water in bottles, you understand'

The waitress is still smiling as she walks past our table. Let's hope she's not French!

***

An elderly man sits alone in the corner of the tea room. Before him lies a cup of coffee, which he sips occasionally, while gazing round the room. I notice he has a brown leather notebook and a smart looking pen, and he is frequently writing notes in the book. He scribbles furiously, and then pauses as though to catch his breath. He continues to look round the room at intervals and I wonder if he is doing the same as I am, recording his observations for the day. I want to leave my sombre table and go ask him what he is writing, but it seems inappropriate, although I know Mum would have done that. She loved to talk to strangers.

***

On the drive home I suddenly feel subdued and low in mood. It all seems so final. Mum and Dad together again and yet, far away from me. There are days I cannot grasp the fact that they are not here, that I will never see them again. My mind can't compute this awful heartbreak and I feel so alone. The reality is, that I am alone in my grief. I have no siblings, no one to share it all with. My heart feels heavy and tired, but I know I just have to go through this feeling to get to the other side. My thoughts bounce, as I wonder just how long it will take to get to the 'other side.' I know it is still early days, but my instinct is telling me that this grief will be with me forever, like the unwelcome visitor to a dinner party. I growl inwardly, hating grief and all that it brings to my shattered life.

At home, I lay on the bed in an emotional heap and cuddle my dog, George, feeling his soft fur within my fingers. I feel strangely comforted by the sight of his deep chestnut eyes that stare at me with such devoted loyalty, and yet, I am aware that this comfort is shortlived, and soon I will feel the intense grief once again. My eyes feel heavy and I pray to whoever is listening that my sleep will be peaceful and my dreams will be happy ones. Just for one night, please.

***

Three things I am grateful for today.

1 My Dad – for all he did for me.

2 My Mum and Dad – great parents and wonderful grandparents.

3 George, my dog and those beautiful brown eyes that melt my heart.

Chapter Fourteen

Saturday 6th May 2023

Today is Coronation Day for the United Kingdom. Yes, today is the day that Prince Charles becomes King Charles after the death of Queen Elizabeth last September. Much like my mother, I can hardly believe the country's beloved Queen has gone. She was just 'always here', smiling broadly with her wonderful, colourful hats, surrounded by her beloved corgis. One day here, the next gone, just like my Mum. Although she was elderly like my Mum, the shock was still huge and left everyone reeling and unsure as to what happens next. That's the problem with death. It changes the status quo, the familiarity, the feeling of steadiness, the comforting safeness of life. Death of a loved one changes everything and we are left living in an unfamiliar world.

The television is on from the early morning so we can soak up the atmosphere of the Coronation Day. The crowds in London gather amid a sea of red, white and blue flags and bunting. Happy, smiling faces fill the television screens, as people from all corners of the world voice their support and love for the new King.

'Isn't it wonderful!' screams an overexcited woman with a deep south American drawl, whilst waving a huge flag, which buries her once the wind changes direction. Her screams of delight are infectious, if not a little ear popping. Sometimes I am grateful for the great British reserve. I'm not sure I could ever scream at any royal or any celebrity for that matter. I think I've only screamed a few times, generally at my children many years ago, when they wouldn't tidy their room. And now, I'm not sure why I did as it always fell on deaf ears.

I watch the day unfold, from the arrival of the prospective King, to the balcony appearance at Buckingham Palace. I haven't done much else today, preferring to immerse myself in watching the TV, avoiding thinking about Mum lying in a souless cemetery, a few miles from where I sit right now. My mother would have loved to watch the Coronation ceremony, in fact, she would have been glued to the TV for hours. She loved to watch and comment on the fashion of the day and of course, she would discuss this with me in graphic detail. This is when I miss her the most. These everyday activities that long for another opinion, another viewpoint. Just someone to talk to.

We decide to go out for dinner, out of pure laziness on my part and I nestle down in the restaurant with my trusty notebook on one hand and my fork in the other. It's funny how no one really notices my writing antics in public. Perhaps they are so immersed in their own life that they don't notice anything unusual in their surroundings. I find that hard to comprehend. As a writer, I am constantly looking for inspiration, ideas and conversations to help me on my own writing journey. My notebook is an extention of myself, my life and my world, and I really cannot be without it on my journey through life, especially now, as I go through the grief process.

***

The restaurant is quiet, presumably as most people are engaged in Coronation parties at home. Barbecues will be fired up, yes, even with the threat of rain that has been lingering all day. In true British tradition, a few cans of beer should help relieve the cool feeling that sweeps in with the grey, rain filled clouds. Just a few lonely souls like myself are enjoying the peace and quiet of a hollow room in a restaurant, the smell of sirloin steak drifting through the dining area.

A young waiter glides round the room as though he is floating on fresh air. I wonder if he is happier with the low number of diners tonight, although his tips will be poor. He smiles at everyone, polite and courteous with all, probably secretly guessing how much he will earn tonight. Doesn't every waiter do that? I know I used to during my brief stint working in a fast food restaurant during my university days.

'Excuse me!'

The silence is broken by a rather stout man sat in the far corner of the room. He perches on the chair at the head of the table, much like a King surveying his peasants. Although I am sure the newly crowned King Charles doesn't look like that when he is having a little late supper in Buckingham Palace.

'Young man. These chips are too salty. Don't you know how bad salt is for us? I have to watch my blood pressure. Please get me some fresh chips with no salt.'

The waiter looks crestfallen as he tries to reason with the customer, explaining that there was no salt added to the chips as that is just not company policy. Eventually he gives up trying and takes the easy option.

'Don't worry sir. I will change the chips immediately and make sure no salt is added. My apologies.'

Just as the waiter hurries away with the 'salt laden' chips, the man's wife arrives back from her visit to the Ladies Room. After a few whispers, it becomes apparant that the perpetrator of the added salt is in fact the man's wife, who sheepishly admits that she added salt while he was not looking. Mr Anti Salt Man turns a rather interesting shade of beetroot and I worry for his blood pressure now. His wife laughs loudly, while tapping him on the back reasurringly, just as the young waiter arrives back with a fresh plate of chips, unsalted of course!

***

I watch the remaining diners as they eat their dinner and I am fascinated by how people eat so differently. Some eat like a frightened dormouse, nibbling at their food while nervously watching all movement in their perimeter. Then there are the guzzlers, who don't care what they look like, as long as the food hits their stomach quicker than an Olympic sprinter. And then there are those that continue to have deep meaningful conversations, while pushing their food around the plate, which usually goes cold by the time they cease talking. As for myself, I eat slowly and mindfully, chewing slowly, savouring every mouthful. Do I do this to be mindful? Nope. I do it to prevent indigestion, another symptom of growing old!

On the journey home I see a flurry of Union Jack flags hanging from windows, trees and even specially erected flag poles made of wooden sticks. The nostalgia brings tears to my eyes, the pride in our country is obvious as we celebrate the new incoming King. I am always aware that there are many who don't like our Royal Family and sometimes I understand their reasoning, with regards to the distribution of wealth. But I am also hugely proud of my country and its history and heritage and I shared these thoughts with my Mum. I remember in the latter stages of her dementia, my Mum excitedly recounted the story of the Queen Elizabeth coming to enjoy afternoon tea the day before. My Mum even told me the colour of the Queen's dress and fancy hat and explained how delicately the Queen had cut the cake for them.

Of course, the Queen hadn't come to afternoon tea with my Mum, and I rather think Mum had seen the Queen recently on the TV and had somehow muddled up the events. But it didn't matter if it was true or not. My Mum was so happy about the Queen's visit and I know she slept peacefully that night with her mind full of wonderful memories (even if they were false.) So, I know how much joy our Royal Family give to the UK, the world and my Mum, and that makes me happy too. Long live the King.

***

Three things I am grateful for today.

1 The British Monarchy. Yes, I like them.

2 Our beloved Queen Elizabeth. RIP.

3 Chips, preferably unsalted.

Chapter Fifteen

Tuesday 9th May 2023

I am stood on a windy platform at my local train station waiting for the 7.37 to London Kings Cross. Tattered Union Jack bunting hangs limply from the station roof, the Coronation now just a distant memory. It's hard to remember that we have a new King as I glance in my purse at the ten pound note proudly showing the late Queen's head. I am suddenly distracted by the shuffling of feet as the crowd of travellers move forward, eager to board the London bound train which is visible in the distance. The rush for a seat is unnecessary, as I board the train unhurried and nestle down into my cocoon for the next three hours, as we leave the peace of the North Yorkshire countryside and head towards the bustling and smoky capital.

***

A smartly dressed young man quickly opens his lap top and proceeds to tap intensely on the keyboard. He glances skyward every few minutes, maybe looking for inspiration, or perhaps he is daydreaming of a place far away from work and responsibilites. I suspect the latter as he takes his phone from the table and calls someone.

'Hi, It's only me. I'm sorry I had to rush out. I had to catch this train.'

'No, I can't get another job. We need the money and London jobs pay better. You know that.'

'No we can't jack in our jobs and travel Europe in our camper van. What a silly idea Eve.'

'See you tomorrow. I do miss you.'

He ends the call, but still clutches his phone, his connection with his beloved Eve. He looks wistfully into the vacuous space in front of him, sighing every few minutes. He pulls his phone close to him and starts scrolling, smiling and gritting his teeth at the same time. I wonder if he is on social media looking at other couples as they travel round Europe in their minimalistic camper vans. I want to lean across to him and whisper 'just do it.' I know it's a decision he has to make for himself, but I pity his tormented mind right now as he battles between his responsibilities and his dreams. I want to tell him that life is too short and we should grab opportunities when we can, but I know that I am currently fuelled by grief and the shock of the fragility of life.

***

I suddenly think of Mum and all the fun things I wish we could have done together. I am awash with sadness, and so I leave the young man scrolling through his phone and dreams and I gaze out of the window hoping for a sign that comforts me in my grief. As the train speeds through the English countryside I am grateful for the expanse of the landscape and the thought of all the wildlife that must live there. Nature is a great healer and I find myself craving the outdoors more and more lately. I check my watch knowing that in a couple of hours the green calming world outside my window will soon be replaced by the grey concrete wilderness of London, and I steel myself for the attack on my delicate senses.

I feel the train alter its speed and I sit upright, suddenly aware that I have been asleep for the last forty minutes. The landscape has indeed changed and my heart sinks looking at the back of soulless industrial units and unkempt back gardens which back onto mainline railways, unaware that they form the welcome sign for visitors approaching London.

Alighting at Kings Cross Station, one of the busiest in the country, I am thrust into a world that fills my heart with dread. I am at home in the tranquil English countryside, surrounded by the morning song of birds and the smells of freshly cut grass. Here, my senses are on overload as I am pushed by impatient travellers, muttering under their breath at my slow pace. I smell everything and nothing, as my nasal cavities reel from all sides, unable to compute exactly what fragrance lingers in the stone cold air. My confused brain tries to understand the multitude of noises that attack from all sides, and in the end it gives up, unable to give meaning to my surroundings. I feel dizzy, unsure and I want to cry. I feel grief, profoundly. I want to be at home, away from everyone and everything.

I am suddenly aware of someone holding my arm, gently and with lightness.

'Are you ok, Miss? You look unsteady there.'

I look round actively blurring out anything in my eyeline, except for the face of an elderly gentleman, aged about 80, who reminds me of my father. It is easy to feel nervous in a busy city particularly for us country girls, but this is different. I know in an instant, this stranger is kind and well meaning and I look at him pleading for help without actually speaking any words.

'It's ok love. Let me sit you down here for a minute. The crowds can be so overwhelming.'

I find myself on a table outside a coffee shop which is unusually quiet. I feel I can breathe again and I turn to say thank you to my guardian angel, but he is gone. Searching the local vicinity I strain my neck trying to see him, but nothing. He is gone. Just like that, he is gone. I search my memory of the past few moments, unsure if I imagined it all. Perhaps we do have a guardian angel who visits us once in a while when we need it the most. I like to think so.

I stand, ready for the next leg of my journey, taking a long, deep breath to sustain my frazzled body. Just a quick glance again on my search for my guardian angel, and just for a moment I think I see him in the throngs of the London crowds. I smile inwardly, silently grateful for kind hearts brought on a gentle breeze, just when I needed it the most.

***

Three things I am grateful for today.

1 Trains. Sometimes slow and never on time, but still an asset.

2 The countryside which always lifts my heart.

3 Guardian angels, there to help us when we least expect it.

Chapter Sixteen

Saturday 27th May 2023

After the buzz of London I am now back home, enjoying the peace and solitude of the North Yorkshire Moors. The rugged landscape stretches out for miles and my eyes strain to see where it ends. Perhaps it doesn't end. Perhaps we are meant to keep searching for the perfect view, the perfect day, the perfect life. Personally, I don't think perfect exists, although my view right now comes very close to perfection.

Today is a day of walking, rambling across the moors and enjoying the freedom of my surroundings, no longer hemmed in by shadowy, sooty walls and ominous concrete blocks that dominate the London streets. The coarse moorland vegetation feels spongy beneath my feet, cushioning my feelings of heaviness. The blue sky sparkles above me, covering me with the comfort of a warm blanket, protecting me from the icy frost that sometimes invades my heart. I place my waterproof cushion down and I sit, content with a flask of hot tea and a round of cheese salad sandwiches wrapped in brown paper and tied with a piece of jute string, just like Mum used to.

Insects crawl excitedly on a rock near my feet, busy, and yet relaxed as they go about their daily activities. I immerse myself in their miniature world, watching them weave among slivers of grass and randomly placed rocks. I wonder if they look up at me, a giant, sat on my throne, intimidating and even threatening. And yet, it couldn't be further from the truth. I have a longing to shrink to their size, to experience their surroundings, to feel their fear and their joy. Is it so different for us humans? We both exist in a world which appears so much bigger than each individual, a world which can sometimes overwhelm us, casting shadows from every angle. And yet, this tiny world of insects seems so simple, so unrushed, uncomplicated, but still with a sense of purpose. I often wonder where the human world went wrong in its bid to achieve a better life for us all, when we are all living through more stress than ever before.

Finishing my lunch, I lay back creating a soft mattress of woodland grasses, feathering my nest and snuggling down with a deep sigh. Cloud watching is the most wonderful, relaxing activity and I think everyone should be encouraged to engage in this form of day dreaming regularly. I always view clouds as pictures and works of art, albeit moving ones. Clouds are more than just white fluffy blobs in the sky. Clouds have meaning, a purpose, a way of speaking to us through the different forms they take throughout their journey. Different hues of white-milky, ghostly, ashen, chalky, snow bleached and even grey, all provide a heartening spectacle to my eyes. I form pictures of each one, seeing faces, figures, animals, mountains and even islands, ever changing like a shapeshifter slithering through different time zones. I reach up eager to touch a cloud so I can caress it and run my fingers through it like downy cotton wool, to feel that softness close to me, to comfort.

I must have fallen asleep. The sky looks heavy and grey and even foreboding, triggering a slight panic in me, although I am unsure why. I feel bereft at the loss of the blue sparkling sky which filled my world with such hope and joy, the clouds providing comfort and respite from my grief. Now, I feel hurried and anxious. My immediate world feels oppressive and out of control and unstable. I jump up from my moorland bed and gather my belongings and quickly head back to the safety of my hotel room. Of course, there is no real threat, merely nature turning the wheel onto the next groove, and yet my body perceives the change in the sky as something to be wary of, something to be scared of.

I have realised that grief can trigger new emotional sensitivities in the mind and body. It's as though everything becomes jumbled, causing confusion and uncertainty. This happens often, and I think it is the body and mind trying to find a new way forward through the maze of grief. Any abrupt and sudden change in the environment around us can make us feel unsteady and unsure. This is so tiring and yet each day I learn something new about my grief. As I lay down praying for a peaceful sleep, I resolve to write a book on my grief experiences one day, but for now, I turn out the light and feel gratitude for my day on the North Yorkshire Moors.

***

Three things I am grateful for today.

1 Nature – all of it!

2 Clouds. So hypnotic and beautiful.

3 The North Yorkshire Moors.

Chapter Seventeen

Sunday 28th May 2023

Right now I am sat on a steam train heading into the Yorkshire countryside. The romantic era of steam never fails to ignite even the most coldest hearts. The vintage carriages with dim, muted lights, the smell of burning coal in the air, the soft 'chug chug' of the train as it slowly makes its way along the tracks. This slow pace of travelling is a world away from our fast motorways and busy town centres, often snarled up with tail to tail traffic. I feel ultra relaxed and have to be aware not to fall asleep with the gentle rocking and repetitive rhythm of this vintage engine.

***

We are sharing our enclosed compartment with other travellers and with courteous greetings and shy smiles completed, we all settle down for the hour journey to our final destination. Nearest the compartment door sit a couple who clearly are dressed for a long hike, laden down with large rucksacks and walking poles. The woman who is dressed in matching waterproof blue jacket and trousers clearly hasn't been on a steam train before.

'It's going slow isn't it Andy? Do you think it's broken?'

'No dear. It's a steam train. It's supposed to go slow.'

Miss 'Never Been On A Steam Train Before' pauses and gazes out of the window. My instinct for reading people tells me that she is thinking deeply about the workings of a steam train. In fact, I can hear her brain working from where I sit.

'Andy, what happens when we come to a steep hill?'

'I guess he will put more coal in the fire and get more power. Don't worry about it Andrea.'

I look across at Andrea who obviously is worried about it and is now biting her lip while frowning.

'Andy, would you like a glass of wine?'

Andy nods his head excitedly and in an instant Andrea is pouring white wine into two plastic glasses, before handing one to her companion. Worry over the steam train's ability to get up hills is long gone, as the happy couple giggle and smile lovingly at each other, while sipping their wine. I am amazed at the swiftness that the wine and glasses were retrieved from the bag and I secretly pray that they don't get too giddy before we reach our destination.

***

In the far corner of our compartment sit an elderly couple, both dressed as though they are on their way to church. I am unsure that any church goers would travel to church on a steam train but I am, as ever, open minded by the actions of the human race. For most of the journey they sit quietly, enjoying the outside views of the passing landscape, while occasionally smiling at each other with a knowing look. A couple of times I notice them glancing disapprovingly at the couple near the door, now on their second glass of chardonnay. I sigh, hoping this doesn't escalate into a drunken steam train event.

Andrea, glass in hand, is starting to look a little tipsy and thankfully her companion decides to reel her in.

'Ok dear, I think you've had enough now.'

Andy sups the rest of the wine and packs the glasses away in the rucksack lying at his feet. His companion sinks back in her seat, smiles to herself, closes her eyes and we all visibly give a sigh of relief. The rest of the journey is spent in peace and we all enjoy the beauty of the Moors from the comfort of our seat.

***

Three things I am grateful for today.

1 Steam trains – the only way to travel.

2 Clever inventors and engineers who create useful things, like trains.

3 My fellow train passengers for making me smile.

Chapter Eighteen

Friday 2nd June 2023

The start of a new month brings some welcome warm sunshine, although I feel a dark cloud in my heart. The further away I get from Mum's passing, the more I feel bubbling panic within me. Will I remember her? Will I forget what she sounds like? I still can't believe that I haven't heard or seen her for three months. I want to scream out that I want, no, I NEED her back. I just can't imagine life without her. Are we ever too old to still want our Mum?

I am aware that we all react differently to grief, and yet the general concensus is that once the funeral is over, the grieving should brush themselves down and move on. I feel so much outside pressure to be constantly smiling and to get on with day to day activities, while inside I'm crumbling and falling apart, and the sun does nothing to help my current mood.

Today we are heading to Lincolnshire for a pre booked event which is a lifelong dream for me. We are taking part in the tour of a wartime Lancaster bomber – the aircraft that was instrumental for the UK in its defeat of the Nazis during the Second World War. I have a passion for history, but especially World War Two, and the Lancaster aircraft is such an iconic plane to any historical war enthusiasts.

Driving through the Lincolnshire countryside is relaxing and healing to the fractured soul. This is one of my favourite counties of England with its long, rolling flat plains of nothingness and hollow emptiness. Periodically, clustered villages appear on our route, and I notice that they all appear timeless, untouched by the modern world. There is something quite therapeutic about these villages that just pop up along endless country roads, and I wonder if the inhabitants feel a sense of safety and security as they huddle in their picturesque country cottages. There is a part of me that wants to stop and seek refuge in one of these cosy houses, sip hot tea out of cracked china cups and enjoy hot buttered crumpets by an open fire. Squinting my eyes at the powerful sun streaming through the car window, perhaps crumpets by a fire is not such a good idea in June.

***

Just an hour later, I am stood at the foot of the giant and magnificent Lancaster Bomber aircraft, slightly apprehensive as our tour guide has explained that we may have to show some agility skills to manoeuvre our way around the aircraft, once inside. I'm not sure I feel particularly agile, but I will make an effort. My fellow travellers on the tour include a retired RAF pilot, a middle aged man with his son who is about eleven years old and an elderly lady who stands quietly in the background as though she is desperate to be consumed into invisibility.

'Dad, why are there no seats on this plane like the one we went on to Lanzarote?'

'Well, Freddy, this plane was used to go to war so it has to be fitted out different. The crew aren't going on holiday so they don't get comfortable seats like we do now.'

'Isn't that unfair though Dad? If they are going to war they should be comfortable before they start fighting.'

'Yes, son. I guess you're right.'

My eyes fall on the elderly lady, who I guess is about eighty years old. A few minutes later she confirms her age as eighty five and I am in awe of her bravery to have signed up for the tour, especially with the forthcoming agility test. She is dressed elegantly and her face portrays a thoughtful and almost sad look. I guess immediately that she has a tale to tell and it isn't long before she shares with the group.

'My father flew in a Lancaster. He was the navigator. He didn't come home. I had to come and see inside the plane, just to feel close to him again.'

The group falls silent and together we bow our head in respect for this great man who gave his life to ensure freedom for his daughter. In that moment of solitude I feel her grief and pain for the father that she never really knew. Even after years have passed, grief is still part of our life, as it secures itself in our every waking moment. As we explore the inside of the giant plane, I feel an emotional bond to this wonderful, brave lady as I watch her cast her eyes on her father's last view of life before he was so cruelly taken away. I wonder about the other crew members and their family they left behind and I realise that no one escapes the monster of grief.

***

I am grateful for the day spent with my fellow travellers, but I am tired, worn down with the emotions of grief. As my head touches the pillow, my cheeks are wet with tears, thinking of all those who also cry tonight, missing loved ones, or fathers that went to war and never returned home.

Three things I am grateful for today.

1 All those that made sacrifices during the second World War.

2 Plane engineers. How clever are they!

3 Peace in our country.

Chapter Nineteen

Saturday 10th June 2023

We are trying to move house and my days are dominated with searching for the perfect property in the ideal location. My inbox is flooded with estate agents begging me to go view their newest property, even though it is outside the specific location that I asked for. Today has been dedicated to viewing potential houses, and so I have made myself look presentable, put a big smile on my face, ready for the repetitive comments of 'Oh, isn't this kitchen spacious? It's wonderful to have a garage AND a double parking space! Look at this neat, well kept garden. Not much for us to do here.'

The reality is that I feel awkward looking round someone else's home. I am an unwelcome intruder gliding round each room, trying to avert my eyes from anything remotely personal. Family photographs adorn the walls, birthday cards fill the window sill, children's drawings pasted on the fridge door and I squirm inside, not knowing where to look. Embarrassed homeowners quickly move that last piece of underwear slung over the radiator, but I smile in acknowledgement, knowing I also do this if I am in a rush to dry wet clothes.

This intrusion into a stranger's life is difficult, but necessary, as we strive to find the right home and so I reassure myself that I am not nosey, but merely deciding if I could live there long term. However, there is a part of me that cannot help but digest the weird habits of human beings, from their choice of decor to the sometimes scary and weird photographs that fill the house. Of course, I would never divulge an address, but there was a particular property we viewed today that made me grateful for the simple life I lead.

***

As soon as we cross the threshold of number 18, my stomach sinks. It is dark and dingy with an air of Victorian England decor, 1890 style. I reassure myself that a tin of magnolia paint would soon change that, but deep down I am already feeling this is not the house for me. I have this romantic notion that the kitchen is the heart of the home. It is a place I envisage myself sat by a fire, with a cat on my knee, reading a book, while my Victoria Sandwich cakes bake in the warm oven. As I enter this kitchen my dreams crumble, or more like, explode into a thousand pieces. I feel like I have stepped onto a film set, AKA Willy Wonka and the Chocolate Factory. An explosion of colour fills the room and I can feel a migraine coming on, even though I don't actually suffer from migraine. The room is silent, no one speaks. There is no smell of freshly baked cakes, just a smell of something that maybe the cat brought in. The owner of this 'enchanting' house speaks first.

'Now I know this is not everyone's cup of tea, but I am really proud of this kitchen. It just makes me feel happy, don't you agree?'

He's right on the first statement. It isn't everyone's cup of tea, or cup of coffee for that matter. In fact, I am struggling to think of anyone in my friendship group who might like this abundance of colour. Reds, yellows, purples, greens are splattered across all four walls, a rather psychedelic background for the vivid red kitchen units, that appear to have red glitter worktops. I say appear, as my eyes are beginning to hurt and my brain is struggling to compute the scene before me. So, to be honest I'm not too sure what colour the kitchen is, as I am feeling a hint of motion sickness. My husband speaks and as always tries to be diplomatic, although he usually fails quite spectacularly at this. Today he does not disappoint.

'Well, it isn't really our colour, to be honest. Although our grandchildren would love it. They are into all this abstract art, paint splattering stuff.'

The room falls silent again. Right now my husband is trying to calculate the cost of ripping out the rainbow kitchen, while the owner stares into space, probably feeling sadness that someone else doesn't appreciate his decor. As for me, I am trying to assess how to exit the house as quick as I can without appearing rude. I don't think quick enough as the home owner is now ushering us out into the hallway and through into the lounge.

The horror comes quicker than I thought as we are standing in a large living room which reminds me of an Amazonian jungle. I feel slightly inadequate and small as I root myself on a large shabby looking sheepskin rug, casting my eye quickly around the room. I am surrounded by plants, a lot of plants. No, not plants. More like trees. Lots of green, bushy trees with so much foliage I can't actually see the walls. I tell myself that it is just decor and I can easily change that. But my sensible head is telling me to be polite and make a quick exit. I take my mobile phone out of my bag, reverting to the old 'family emergency' excuse.

'Oh, I'm dreadfully sorry but I have just received an urgent text from my daughter and we have to go now. Family emergency, you understand.'

***

Neither of us speak as we head to the nearest coffee shop for a caffeine fix to calm our frazzled nerves. Buying a house is going to be more difficult than I thought, but this piece of red velvet cake is definitely helping to reinstate a sense of calm to my nervous state. It is at times like this that I wish desperately my Mum and Dad were here. I long to have their valuable opinion on what house to buy, and more than anything I want them to walk through the door of my new house.

Any way tomorrow we start all over again. Please let tomorrow's house be that perfect one.

***

Three things I am grateful for today.

1 That I am able to move house when I fancy a change.

2 Quirky people who make me smile.

3 My ability to think of a good excuse to get out of a difficult situation.

Chapter Twenty

Sunday 18th June 2023

Today is Father's Day, a day I have grown to dislike intensely. In the previous few weeks I have rushed past the abundance of cards in the shops that only highlight the fact I have no father anymore. I think of millions of others like me, and wonder how they get through these days, when they are constantly reminded of the loss of a loved one. I am, by my nature, a very nostalgic person. I think often about days gone by, I can recall detailed memories without too much thought, and I often 'feel' a huge emptiness in my stomach, knowing I will never get those days back.

So today, I will try and avoid all Father's Day reminders, enjoying a quiet Sunday with my dog George and my husband. A walk in the countryside is always the best way to start a day, even a day tinged with sadness and so I head off to one of my favourite walks, deep in the Yorkshire countryside. Dreams of a quiet walk without interruption quickly disappear, as I seem to have joined a myriad of others, probably also trying to escape the Father's Day hype.

***

I see a tall, red cheeked man of about sixty years old approaching me at great speed. I put my head down hoping he ignores me but alas, he speaks, puffing and panting like a worn out steam train.

'Morning. Have you seen a sheep?'

I glance round, catching sight of at least fifty sheep in the field next to the footpath I am stood on.

'Ermmm, what colour is it?' I try to look interested, but I know I am failing miserably.

'White'

I smile weakly, while gesturing over the grey stone wall.

'Nah, they're not my sheep, are they?

The truth is, I have never met this man before and I certainly haven't met his sheep, and so I am at a loss how to answer. To be honest, I think all sheep look the same, but I know I will get pilloried for saying that. Mr 'Sheep Man' doesn't seem to notice or care about my indifference and he walks off, whistling to himself, or maybe he is whistling for his lost sheep. I feel there is a story there somewhere, but I carry on my walk, secretly hoping the lost sheep is found quickly.

Just ahead I notice a couple sat in front of a wall. They are engrossed in each other and the rather fabulous spread of food before them. As it isn't quite lunchtime, I guess that this is 'brunch' and I am intrigued by the rather delicious array of food neatly laid on a red checked table cover. Matching red napkins are spread across their laps as the woman starts to pour hot coffee from a Thermos. I know for a fact it is coffee as I can smell the tantalising aroma of freshly ground beans as she pours the chestnut elixir into two delicate china cups. I think back to our picnic last week as we hiked on the moors, the cheese sandwiches wrapped in brown paper, served with a bag of Seabrook crisps, cheese and onion flavour. Stewed tea was then poured into the plastic cups that come with the flasks, the ones that hold a thimbleful of liquid that you have to drink quickly before it gets cold. A bashed up orange was our dessert, before wiping our hands with a piece of kitchen roll. I notice the 'Picnic' couple enjoying a plump and colourful fresh fruit salad from blue floral bowls and I make a mental note that I must go shopping for some decent picnicware. This is the second time this year that I have been envious of a traveller's picnic. There must be a subliminal message in there somewhere.

***

My stomach starts to rumble in reaction to the delicious feast it has just witnessed, and I reach into my dog walking bag to retrieve a flattened cereal bar that I think has been living in the depth of my bag since last Christmas.

'It will be ok' I say to myself as I peel back the enticing orange wrapper, desperately trying to get excited by the crumbled mess I see before me. I greedily eat it, while imagining it is something delectable from the local deli. Of course, my imagination isn't that good and I feel like I've eaten a piece of cardboard the dog has chewed. My pace quickens as I head back home, hoping my husband has made me a bacon sandwich.

***

I see a family playing in a local park. Mum, Dad and two young children are enjoying fun time playing football. I suddenly notice an older couple join them, screams of delight and laughter rings loud from the group. I realise they have their parents with them. Three generations together, enjoying and celebrating Father's Day. I am transfixed by the scene. There is a part of me that wants to join in, to feel the warmth of family love once again, to shout 'Dad' and see his smile as he plays football with my children. It is a scene I go through many times, to try relive it, to experience that warm, fuzzy feeling yet again. But it is lost, gone forever. There will be no more playing football with my Dad. It hurts, really hurts, and I leave the happy family, with a hint of envy for what they are experiencing right now. I turn back to watch them one final time and I long to shout, 'enjoy every moment because it won't be here forever.' Of course, I remain silent and I walk home, feeling the grief as it moves through my body.

Happy Father's Day, Dad, wherever you are.

***

Three things I am grateful for today.

1 Picnics in the summer – although I must try harder.

2 Watching families play happily.

3 My Dad. The best Dad ever.

Chapter Twenty-One

Tuesday 4th July 2023

A new month and I can hardly believe it is July already. The months seem to be flying past. Traditionally, July in the UK is known as strawberry and Wimbledon month, and coincidentally my husband has managed to get two tickets for the Wimbledon Tennis Championships. As I write this, he is on a train speeding towards London with his brother, in anticipation of watching some world class tennis over the next couple of days.

Yes, I had the chance to go, but since Mum's death I have shied away from crowds, feeling overwhelmed and anxious at the thought of being hemmed in by hundreds of bodies. And so, I opt for a quiet few days at home helped by the arrival of one of my dearest friends who is staying with me for a few days. We are spending the day in my local town, shopping, drinking coffee and, of course, observing real life people for my journal.

***

A man in his fifties, casually dressed, sits on a bench outside Marks and Spencers. He is surrounded by shopping bags of various shapes and sizes that seem to dwarf his body. He clutches a coffee in a red takeaway cup, staring wistfully into the crowds. I wonder what he is thinking, or is he thinking at all? He reminds me of my own father who was chief bag carrier for my mother during her weekly shopping trips. I remember only too well the same vague expression, that look of resignation and acceptance. No complaining, no moaning, just that quiet willingness to support one's partner.

I look again at him and I notice his facial expression has suddenly changed. At first I cannot see the reason for this, but then I notice a tall, blond haired lady approaching him from the street. He smiles widely, his eyes rooted on the woman in question. She puts her arm around him and he offers her the coffee cup in his hand. She takes it, sips and grimaces, then laughs. I deduce that the coffee was cold, probably due to the fact that he has been sat there for sometime. They exchange words, smiling and laughing, she nods her head and he stands, clutching all the surrounding bags. She offers her arms out as a gesture to carry some of the bags, but he waves her away, smiling. She looks up at him adoringly and puts her arm through his bag laden arm and they walk off together. From this tiny snippet I concur that many men secretly enjoy their role as bag handler for their wives. This makes me smile knowing that my father spent many 'happy' hours carrying bags for my mother because he loved her, and it was his way of showing it. Love doesn't always have to be hearts and flowers. Sometimes love is shown through the most mundane every day activities.

***

I drift into a Marks and Spencer store and I can't help listening in to a conversation between two well dressed, elderly ladies. who are clutching lingerie. I promise this is not eavesdropping but essential journalling of everyday life as presented by ordinary, everyday people! The taller lady speaks without lowering her voice.

'Thank goodness for Marks and Spencer underwear. You know where you are with them.'

'Oh yes, Barbara. Gone are the days of frilly, skimpy knickers. I need my big knickers now to keep my kidneys warm.'

'And to be honest, no one cares now what I wear under my dresses. As long as I look decent, in case I have to go to hospital, then that's good enough for me.'

'Oh yes. Our mothers were right, Barbara. Always wear nice, clean knickers in case you get taken away in an ambulance.'

They giggle like a pair of schoolgirls and are still giggling quietly as they approach the till with their purchases. I can't help smiling as my beloved mother also said the same thing to me. Quickly exiting the queue, I head for the lingerie department, with a sudden desire to buy some decent underwear, feeling that my Mother is watching over me as I do.

***

Enjoying a coffee upstairs in the same store, I am overwhelmed by all the different conversations going on in such a small space. It fills me with such warmth that life and people can be so varied and so interesting, if only we would stop to notice and listen.

A young girl is colouring in a picture while her mother sips a frothy coffee, enjoying a few moments quiet time. This is soon broken by the young girl's cry.

'What's wrong Emmi?' the mother asks with a concerned look.

Emmi sobs uncontrollably, staring at her tiny hand.

'Emmi, Tell Mummy what is wrong.'

Emmi gasps for breath and looks up at her mother with tear filled eyes.

'Mummy, I broke the red crayon and I NEED the red crayon!'

In just a few minutes Emmi has taught us what it is like to view life through the eyes of a child, what's important and how important it is. I long for a life where my biggest stress is breaking a red crayon, and I make a note that I must try to reduce my stress and not to get anxious about the little things.

***

Walking back to my car which is parked in a council owned car park, I hear raised voices coming from the car parked next to mine. A well dressed man in his forties is arguing with a car parking attendant, who appears to be writing out a parking ticket.

'Look, I'm only ten minutes over my time. I left my cash card in a shop and I had to go back for it. That's why I'm late!'

The pleading of the car owner seems to be falling on deaf ears, literally, as there is no response from the traffic warden. Nothing. This obviously riles the car owner who is now shouting obscenities at the parking attendant who is now sticking the parking ticket to the window of the car. Having completed his job, he slowly walks away, ignoring the pleas of the car owner. For a moment I wonder if the car park attendant is actually deaf as he seems oblivious to what is going on. And then, I see it. A wry smile appears on his face, a proud look of a person who enjoys his job and won't be intimidated by any angry motorists. The battle is won and I am so concerned I could be next, that I decide to put an alarm on my phone warning me when my parking time is due to expire. I realise that the battle with a car parking attendant is not one I want to enter, and is certainly one I will never win.

***

Later, at home, I am remembering a lovely day shopping and as always, learning about human nature and what makes us feel stressed or calm. My thoughts return to Emmi and I pray that she has a replacement red crayon to ease her pain. Although, understanding a little about children, I actually think that she probably has forgotten all about the red crayon and has focused her attention on something else. A yellow crayon perhaps?

***

Three things I am grateful for today.

1 My husband who will carry all the shopping bags.

2 Marks and Spencer underwear. It is the best!

3 The innocence of children. Don't let them grow up too soon!

Chapter Twenty-Two

Monday 10th July 2023

Today I'm at the hospital with my husband who is undergoing routine tests on possible issues with his prostate. He was told that prostate issues are quite common in men of a certain age, but this still does not alleviate the anxiety and worry that I feel right now, as we cross the threshold of the hospital.

The hospital is, of course, very busy. People congregate in the bright reception area, eager to find out where they need to be, worried faces plentiful. We are directed to follow the 'yellow' line on the floor until we reach our destination. Anxious or not, I can't help but sing 'Follow The Yellow Brick

Road' to myself as we follow the 'important' yellow line, marching endlessly down long, dreary corridors, which all look surprisingly the same.

The truth is, I hate hospitals, especially this one. My last visit here was when Mum was alive. I push the thought to the back of my mind. Today is all about my husband and his peeing frequency. Memories of Mum will have to wait.

***

We reach our destination. A small compact waiting room, windowless and souless. Posters on the wall reminding visitors of the symptoms of prostate cancer and the urgency to get things checked. I sigh. Yes, that's why we are all here. I am the only female in the waiting room, apart from the nursing staff who are friendly and reassuring. I sit opposite an elderly man reading a book. He is concentrating so hard, I can imagine he is absorbing every single word, comma and full stop. The book he is reading is one of my favourites. Munich by Robert Harris. I consider talking to him about the book but I hesitate, thinking that maybe this isn't the right time. I notice he hasn't turned a page in over five minutes and I wonder if he is reading at all. Maybe it's his way of blocking out the world while he has to deal with health issues. I wish his wife could be here, to support him in his hour of need. I wonder if he has a wife. The thought of it all makes me feel incredibly sad, and I wish I could have a magic wand and wave away all the pain and worry he is going through.

***

Soon he is called in to the examination room and we are alone. I try to talk to my husband, but it is clear he wants to be alone with his thoughts and his worries. I respect his feelings and I pick up a gardening magazine which lies on the table next to me. I contemplate how different men are from women, in that they don't talk about their worries and fears as we do, preferring instead to ruminate and stay silent. I think of my own father who kept his illness to himself, preferring to act as though nothing was wrong. There is a tiny part of me that still holds a sliver of anger towards him for doing this, for shutting me out when I could have helped him. He died suddenly and I often think it could have been prevented. If only I had known, I could have changed the outcome. My life has been full of 'if onlys' but this particular one still breaks my heart even now, ten years after his sudden death.

My deeply disturbing thoughts are broken as I hear my husband's name being called and I see him disappear into a corner room with a momentary backward glance and a wry smile. I whisper 'good luck' just in time to hear the door close. I take a long swig of water, eager to find something to do. Remembering I have just downloaded Scrabble on my phone, I quickly log in and start the first of many games, desperate to block out my anxiety. It works. I am constantly beaten at Scrabble by the computer and I start to question whether it is fixed. Am I really that bad at Scrabble? And why am I always constantly awarded the difficult letters, the Q, the X. I find myself pleading to the phone to give me a little leeway as I am having a difficult day. My prayers are answered as I actually win one game. OK, I played ten games in all, but I was stressed and playing under pressure. I put my phone back in my bag, annoyed with my lack of word knowledge, just as my husband comes out of the consulting room. He looks a bit green round the face, but otherwise okay.

***

We start to make our way back to the car for our homeward journey and I stop at the car park paying machine. A lady appears nervous and struggling to make sense of how to pay. After watching her for a couple of minutes, I cannot hold back any longer.

'Are you OK? Do you need any help?'

'Oh yes, how kind. I just can't seem to work this machine.'

I help her navigate the pay machine, aware of her shaking hands.

Two minutes later she is smiling, clutching her ticket in her hand.

'Thank you so much. It's been quite a day.' She pauses. 'You see, my daughter had her first child this morning, a little girl and I just can't think straight with all the excitement. It's just a miracle. Life IS good.'

***

On our way home I think of the new grandmother, flushed, red cheeks, filled with pride and a deep love for her daughter and new granddaughter. I think of the circle of life, the births, the deaths. So much emotion that can be overwhelming at times and yet, we carry on, hopeful that the good times will, in fact, replace the bad times.

FOOTNOTE – My husband did receive good news about his prostate problem. Nothing to worry about. Life IS good.

***

Three things I am grateful for today.

1 Doctors, nurses and all who work in hospitals.

2 My husband's good health.

3 New life.

Chapter Twenty-Three

Saturday 5th August 2023

Today we are in Lincolnshire again at an air show which also incorporates a 1940's theme. I enjoy reading and experiencing anything related to the 1940's, and so I am looking forward to the day. I have always had my feet firmly rooted in nostalgia, some would call it the 'good old days.' It is a phrase my Mum used a lot, and she liked nothing better than to reminisce, poring over old photos and listening to songs from a bygone era. Since she passed away I appear to have taken on a deeper meaning of nostalgia, and I find myself craving any snippets of the past. As the great singer Doris Day once sang, 'gonna take a sentimental journey, gonna set my heart at ease.'

Delving into the past gives me that warm, cosy and safe feeling, and somehow I feel closer to my Mum when I am locked in this mood.

So, today I am completely enveloping myself in the 1940's, an era that was difficult to live through, but the sense of community and supporting each other was so strong, that I mourn for those days that we don't have now. The weather isn't great. Typical British summer weather, drizzling one minute, then brilliant sunshine the next. The crowds at the air show are not phased by the unpredictable weather, which again, is typically British. Umbrellas emblazoned with Union Jacks and Spitfires are everywhere and I have just seen a large black umbrella with Winston Churchill's face proudly stamped on it.

***

The man standing under Churchill's beaming face, complete with cigar is a rather portly man, dressed in black suit and a 1940's Homburg hat. I do a double take. He is the image of the great man himself,

Winston Churchill. I can't help staring at the uncanny resemblance and I am transfixed by the way he moves, his walk, his mannerisms and facial expressions. The man in question catches my eyes, smiles and promptly performs a V for Victory sign with his right hand, an action associated with the Prime Minister during the Second World War. I return the smile, blush a little, and am overwhelmed with a feeling of sadness that my Mum isn't here to experience the day. She would have loved it. Deep breath Susanna. Enjoy the day, as your Mum would want you to.

***

Because of the unpredictable weather the air displays are cancelled, which is disappointing, but understandable. Instead we are treated to a taxi-run by the great and powerful Lancaster, the same plane I visited a couple of months ago. Listening to the deafening roar of the engines, I feel emotion on another level, as I think of the young airmen that sacrificed their lives in order to ensure freedom from tyranny for our country. The crowds are similarly entranced by the Lancaster as it taxies down the runway, with all eyes transfixed on this powerful metal beast.

***

A lady in front of us is resplendent in her 1940's suit, classic hairstyle and bright red lipstick. She even wears stockings with a black line painted up the back. Very 1940's. She turns to her partner who is smartly dressed in an 1940's RAF uniform.

'Robert, dear. I am in need of a cup of tea. Shall we retire to the tea room?'

Robert nods his head, retaining his proud stance as an RAF officer for the day. They turn to head for the aforementioned tea room and I catch her parting words.

'Robert. Just because we are reenacting the 1940's today doesn't mean we have to ration ourselves, does it?'

'No dear. Does this mean you would like a slice of Victoria Sandwich cake?'

'Oh Robert. You know me so well.'

Her nostalgic floral perfume wafts in my face as they pass, and I thank God for men like Robert who understands a woman's need for cake with a cup of tea in the afternoon. As I lose sight of them in the crowd I secretly hope there is enough Victoria Sandwich cake left for me when I go to the tea room, as I have now developed a strong craving for that delicious light sponge cake.

***

At the next sign of rain, we head indoors to the large plane hangar where we can hear wonderful sounds of 1940's dance music. We enter to see a group of dancers enjoying some swing dancing to the great delight of the crowds that have gathered, also escaping the rain. I manage to find a seat next to an elderly lady of about eighty who is dressed in a stunning royal blue 1940's suit, complete with a matching hat, adorned with a feather. She is tapping her feet to the music and singing unrestricted, oblivious to whoever is watching her. I love her sense of freedom, enjoying the music and the lively atmosphere. The joy on her face is clear. She is having the time of her life. I find myself tapping my feet too, in unison with her. The 'Blue Suit' lady is obviously enjoying herself, but I wonder if she realises the joy she is giving to others.

As the music slows down into a ballad number, she starts swaying from side to side and looks lost in her thoughts. I wonder what she is thinking about, the memories, the good times, the past? Suddenly, one of the dancers approaches her with an outstretched hand. She smiles at him and stands gingerly to her feet. This is her moment. With skill and grace the 'Blue Suit' lady is twirled around the dance floor to an ecstatic audience. Her dance partner treats her with kindness and compassion, not rushing and not too much spinning. Her face is a picture of happiness, lit by a light that seems only to focus on her. She is living in another world, another life, dancing as though she is twenty again. I am mesmerised by what I am witnessing, as are many others in the audience and for a moment I think of my Mum who loved to dance, especially to 1940's tunes.

***

As I leave, I glance back at the lady in blue who is enjoying all the attention from the crowd, eager to congratulate her on her wonderful dancing. For a second I think she looks like a young girl, her face unlined by age or hardship. Her smile is natural, her eyes twinkle and she walks with the grace of a ballerina. Her advancing age is irrelevant. All that matters in that moment is a joyous experience, one that she, and I, will never forget. It was a good day today. Nostalgia really can bring calm and peace to a grieving heart.

***

Three things I am grateful for today.

1 Winston Churchill. He fought hard for our freedom.

2 Nostalgia. It gives me a warm cosy feeling.

3 The older generation. They have so much to offer and we should appreciate them more.

Chapter Twenty-Four

Sunday 13th August 2023

The sun peeks around the bedroom curtains as I open my eyes to yet another day without seeing Mum. She is the first thing I think about on waking, and just for a split second I plan my next visit to her, before quickly realising those days are now gone. It's funny how our brains work, almost fooling us into thinking all is okay, and then the crushing realisation that everything is not okay.

Today we are going to a local country show. I love country shows. A hub of wild and wonderful farm animals, delicious food stalls, craft and produce hosted in large weather-worn marquees, and visitors enjoying a relaxing day in the sunshine. This particular show is rather more interesting than most as I have entered a photograph in the photography category and a Christmas tree made entirely from buttons in the handicrafts section. Sometimes I don't know why I enter shows as I get a little stressed, hoping my exhibits will live up the standard of the other competitors, but something drives me to at least try.

***

Anyway, my entries are safely in the craft tent awaiting the judges decision and we start wandering round the rest of the show. First stop is the animal section where a host of animals wait patiently in pens, while the judge, looking fetching in a bleached white coat, frowns and smiles, whilst revealing no hint of who the lucky winners are. A young girl of about ten asks the question we all want to ask.

'But Mummy, all those sheep look the same. How does he know which is the best sheep?'

'Well, Alicia. He is an expert on sheep and so he knows what to look for when he is judging.'

'I would give them all a winning rosette as they are all pretty and cute.'

Alicia most definitely speaks for us all in that moment. All the sheep are indeed pretty and cute.

***

We decide to move on and visit the craft and produce tent to look at all the entries. If I'm been honest I am desperate to know if I have won a prize for my own efforts. I make my way through the hoards of people in the tent who obviously are as desperate as I am. It feels like an unsupervised football match, as I struggle to make headway to the tables where I know my entries are waiting for me. I give up trying at one point, but then the determined me is triggered back into life and I manage to squeeze past a couple of ladies who are sauntering at a snails pace. I attract a haughty look from one of them, but at this stage I don't care. My mission is to discover if I have won a prize. My eyes look forward and there it is in the distance. My beloved button Christmas tree. And what is that in front of it? I spy a bright red card. Excitedly, I accelerate and quickly make my way to the table. FIRST PRIZE! Really? Yes, first prize for my red and green button tree that took me an eternity to create. I stand by my prized tree, eager to savour the moment of victory. Two ladies approach me, smiling broadly. Oh yes, the same two ladies who I squeezed past just a few moments ago. I hold my breath, wondering what is coming next.

'Oh, this Christmas tree is so lovely. Are you the person who made it?'

Smiling widely and proudly, I confirm I am indeed the creator of the tree.

'Wonderful. Could you be a love and explain how you made it? I really want to make one for myself.'

***

And so, I start explaining the intricacies of making a Christmas tree with buttons, my pride growing and growing as I suddenly feel like I have achieved something truly wonderful that other people want to share in. After ten glorious minutes proudly detailing my work of art, I look up to see an captivated audience of about a dozen people, all entranced with my method of creating a Christmas tree with buttons.

How wonderful is it, that sharing something so simple, can create a feeling of community and togetherness. I wonder how different the world would be if we all shared knowledge on a regular basis. Many years ago skills and crafts used to be shared among communities, but this is now a lost art as our world advances quickly, leaving behind old values and traditions.

Enjoying my short burst with stardom, the crowds quickly disperse and my little Christmas tree sits on its own, once again. Taking one more photo of it, like a proud parent, I head for the photographic section to find, to my amazement, that I have also won first prize for my photo of George dressed in red, white and blue

Union Jack bunting. The appropriately named class is 'Jubilee' and I have to say I am enjoying this process of winning with my creations. They say creativity makes you feel good and I absolutely concur with that.

***

I take a photo of my winning entry and am suddenly aware of an elderly gentleman smiling at my photo.

'Is that your dog?'

I smile proudly and confirm it is, waiting for the questions about my photographic technique.

'I had a dog once.'

The man, having said his piece, turns and is soon lost in the crowded throng still in the marquee.

***

I smile inwardly, hoping that my photo brought some joy to him in some small way. On the way home,

I visualise a host of people planning how to make Christmas trees with buttons inspired by my effort. Today has been a good day of sharing and engaging with strangers. Sometimes we can find joy in the unexpected little things.

***

Three things I am grateful for today.

1 Country shows – so much fun.

2 Animals, especially sheep.

3 My ability to create things, especially Christmas trees made with buttons.

Chapter Twenty-Five

Tuesday 5th September 2023

Right now, I am in a queue clutching my passport, trying to leave the country. 'Trying' is the crucial word here as the queue is never ending and we have already missed our scheduled Eurotunnel train. We are, once again on our way to Switzerland for a few weeks, to see our wonderful friends and to enjoy the stunning Swiss scenery. I am feeling happier about our travels this time, as I am slowly coming to terms with the loss of my Mum. Grief is still an unwelcome visitor, but I am learning how to manage it more effectively. Yes, sometimes this means I am deliberately distracting myself from thinking about it, but that's okay. We have to do whatever we can do to cope with the overwhelming grief.

A few hours later we are on our way and heading through France. It is an absolute joy driving through France with their wide, open roads and welcoming service areas that sell the most delicious food, unlike our own British service stations. We have arrived at a service area, and as my husband goes in first to select his breakfast, I am left walking our dog George on a suitable grassy area with considerable shade from the abundance of trees. The shade is needed as the sun is unforgiving today and it is incredibly hot. George is extremely slow at 'doing his business' as he likes to pick the perfect spot, which can take time. While walking him I am thinking what French delicacies I might choose for my breakfast. My stomach rumbles, thinking of the hot croissants and mouth watering baquettes that await me inside the service area food court.

***

Suddenly out of nowhere, a girl aged about ten appears from behind a tree. She is holding her mother's hand and also holding a bright blue dog lead which connects to a small fluffy white dog. Sadly I do not know the breed, but it is cute and cuddly with the brightest black eyes I have ever seen.

I say 'hello' hoping she is English and can understand me. She is French, but of course she speaks good English, much to my shame as I can only speak a few words in French.

'Hello to you too. You are English?'

'Yes, I am. Je m'appelle Susanna and my chien George.'

She smiles and then giggles, looking up at her Mother. I am unsure what she finds funny, but I have a feeling it is me (moi.)

'It is okay English lady Susanna and George. I can speak perfect English. You English are not very good at speaking French are you?'

She giggles again and I am aware I am blushing. I explain I am on holiday and I tell her I love her country very much, especially the food.

'Thank you English lady. I have been to England once, but I did not like your noisy roads or your sandwiches made with bread that is hard and curly at the ends.'

Her mother smiles awkwardly at me and I sigh. How can I argue with that?

'Have a nice holiday English lady!'

***

And in a moment she has disappeared with her mother and her cute little dog and I am left feeling embarrassed at the thought of visitors to the UK, grimacing at our curly sandwiches and noisy roads. I make a pledge to myself in this moment that I will never make a sandwich with inferior bread again.

Finally, my husband returns with his delicious breakfast and I am in the queue at a food stall called Paul's, praying that someone speaks English well enough for me to get my baguette of choice. I speak too soon. I try to explain what I would like to buy, but I am faced with head shakes from the rather glamorous, non-English speaking assistant. I turn to Plan B and start pointing like a conductor at the Royal Philharmonic Orchestra at the vast array of food on display, pointing in particular to a cheese salad baguette. Someone behind me giggles and I fear I have morphed into the crazy English woman in just a matter of minutes. What is left of my dignity I use graciously, and so I turn round to see the young French girl with her mother, but without the dog. I smile and they smile back. I grab my much needed baguette, clutch it close to my chest and run back to the car, embarrassed, hot and determined that next time I visit France I will know a few more words other than hello and goodbye.

Finishing my delicious baguette, we head back out onto the empty French motorway, where I am suddenly grateful for non-noisy roads. Thank you

France for putting up with my crazy English antics and thank you for the best sandwiches ever!

***

Three things I am grateful for today.

1 French roads. Honestly the best I've ever driven on.

2 French baquettes. Seriously good.

3 My French teacher telling me I would never be fluent in French. She wasn't wrong!

Chapter Twenty-Six

Friday 15th September 2023

Settled in Switzerland and feeling relaxed, I am eager to make the most of every minute I am here. My last trip to Switzerland was full of sadness and grief and I am determined this visit will not be the same. Seeing our wonderful Swiss friends again brightens my mood and I can feel a certain lightness in my heart as we catch up with each other's news. It all seems so different from our last visit when my grief was overwhelming. Visiting this beautiful country always brings me joy and this particular visit seems more poignant than any other. Perhaps my deep feeling of gratitude is allowing me to really 'be here' in the present moment. I feel lucky and blessed to be in

Switzerland again and my heart feels so at home here. I wonder if they will let me stay here forever. Perhaps I could hide in a mountain hut, with just the sound of bells waking me every morning. How wonderful would that be? I often think I should have been Swiss. I am so at peace here, with the landscape and the people. Oh well, enough day dreaming. Back to reality and on this beautiful sunny day with cloudless blue skies, we are heading to the village of Iseltwald which lies on the shore of stunning Lane Brienz. It is one of my favourite Swiss villages.

The weather and beauty of this tiny village bring out the tourists, and I notice two coaches already parked up in the market square car park. Hoping it won't be too busy is perhaps optimistic, but unphased, we head for the shore of the lake which is cocooned protectively by the powerful mountains. Immediately, we notice a large group of tourists gathering at the edge of the lake taking numerous photos of their loved ones and friends. Listening in to their conversations I conclude that these tourists are from all over the world, all here to appreciate the beauty of this Swiss landscape.

***

I position myself next to an American couple, who are attempting to take the same photo as myself, albeit with the largest camera I have ever seen.

'Darlene! Stop fidgeting with your hair and let me take the godamn photo!'

'Cameron dear. I just want to get the perfect photo for the kids.'

'Darlene, honey. You are perfect.'

The air seems to hold its breath as we wait for Darlene's response.

'Oh Cammie, you say the nicest things. What would I do without you?'

Photos are taken of the lovely Darlene and we decide to move on, but not before a parting comment from Cameron.

'Now, can we get back to the hotel as this mountain air is giving me a headache and I need a beer.'

***

Darlene and Cameron make their way to the car park to head back for their headache relieving beer and we walk along the shoreline looking for a quieter spot.

Firmly routed on a wooden bench overlooking the lake, it is time to relax and enjoy the beauty of the surrounding landscape. In my opinion views like these should be savoured with silence, allowing the peace to drift over a tired mind and body. The water laps gently on the shore creating a hypnotic rhythm that is lulling me to sleep. My heavy eyes close as I feel my breathing slows down. The peace and solitude is welcomed into an exhausted body that has been in a constant battle for the last few months. I feel I am drifting gently to sleep and I am happy with that. In fact, I am enjoying being in this whole dreamy process away from the noisy world.....

***

'Darlene, now PLEASE can we get back to the hotel?'

'Cammie, I need to take some photos of this beautiful place. I mean, honey, take a look at the colour of this water.'

I squirm in my seat at the interruption and float open my eyes to see Darlene paddling in the shallow edges of the lake. Her travel companion Cameron is stood a few yards away from the water, cautiously, making sure his feet don't get wet.

'Cammie, baby. Just look at the colour! It matches what I'm wearing.'

'Oh Darlene. It sure does.'

Darlene is not wrong. Her turquoise blue silk dress blends in perfectly with the delicate hues of Lake Brienz. She reminds me of a mermaid hovering on the edge of the waterline, trying to decide if she should stay on land or dive into the watery lake. There is silence. The cool, fresh air hovers like a whisper on a cloud. Nothing moves. I cast my eyes on the American couple who are completely transfixed by the colour of the water. They say time stands still when you are enjoying a perfect moment in life, and right now I do believe Darlene and Cammie are having THEIR moment. The cool beer waiting for Cammie at the hotel is long forgotten. I wonder if they will remember this moment when they return to real life? Switzerland certainly has a way of penetrating into the hardest of hearts with its dramatic beauty and gentle peace, that any traveller can't help but fall in love with.

The peace is suddenly broken by the sound of Darlene squealing at the sight of a small duck which seems to have taken quite a shine to her. As she frantically waves her arms about like a windmill, Cammie (and myself) are laughing at the extraordinary scene of a tall, statuesque blond woman trying to run away from a solitary duck, while wading in water trying not to get her dress wet. She fails miserably as her frantic splashing causes a surge of water to soak the front of her dress. Cammie laughs uncontrollably and I get the feeling it is the funniest thing he has seen all year. I have to admit, I am struggling to stifle my giggles. Darlene exits from the lake, her pride a little battered, although her perfect coiffured hair is still in place.

With a protective arm around his beloved Darlene, Cammie gently guides them both back to the village centre and probably straight back to the hotel to get dried and to pick up that cold beer, finally.

***

I witness the 'rogue' duck swimming gracefully along the lake edge, emitting the loudest quacking noises I have ever heard. There was a little cheeky part of me that thought for a moment that the duck was actually laughing. But of course, that wouldn't be true – or would it?

As the sun sets over the lake that night, I smile and feel at peace. I enjoyed my day at Iseltwald and more importantly I had enjoyed 'meeting' Darlene and Cammie for providing the entertainment for the afternoon, not forgetting the duck who was, by now, long gone across the lake, probably on the hunt for more interesting tourists.

After a cup of Swiss hot chocolate at our chalet, I feel that the peaceful world of sleep will be a restful one for me tonight. Some days are just made more wonderful by the people in our lives that cross our path unexpectedly. And as my head touches the pillow, I silently say thank you to those I met today. Quack Quack!

***

Three things I am grateful for today.

1 The beautiful Swiss village of Iseltwald.

2 Darlene and Cammie – who fell in love with Switzerland as I did.

3 Wildlife, ever constant, helping heal the pain of grief.

Chapter Twenty-Seven

Thursday 5th October 2023

We arrived back home from Switzerland just a few days ago and we are faced with an abrupt return to real life. Today may or may not be a difficult day. Twelve months after our dog George was diagnosed with an aggressive cancer, he is back in the veterinary hospital for full body scans and tests to see if he has finally beaten the big C. The past year has been one of nervousness and also joy, as we try and give George the best year of his life, while he is still with us. I can't pretend that I haven't felt huge anxiety, watching every move he makes and every breath he takes. (Yes, that appears to be a famous line from a song by the Police – funny how I remembered that as I sit here writing in my journal!)

For all the anxiety over George's health, we have remained positive and hopeful for a good and successful recovery. But today is the day when we find out if our positivity has been justified. As we walk in the door of the veterinary hospital, I glance down at my beloved George and silently will him to be okay. If love alone could save him, then I know he will be well. I love him so much, I often feel my heart will burst.

We sit quietly in the waiting room, drinking tea to calm the nerves and soothe the dry mouth caused by this overwhelming anxiety. It is busy in the hospital. Nurses come and go, calling in various animals through into the main body of the hospital. Pet owners look anxious, tired and drained and I feel I am in a special club, all united by the fear of what comes next for our precious pets.

***

A woman aged about seventy sits opposite us clutching a small white dog in her arms, wrapped in a pastel coloured blanket. I can see two brown eyes peeking out from behind the woollen cocoon. Eyes that dart from side to side, anxious, nervous, too scared to move. I try smiling at the owner of the white fluffball, but her thoughts are taking her away to another place, far away from here, I am guessing. I am in total agreement with her, as I too start to wish I was somewhere else. I wonder if she is also waiting for news that will determine if her dog has reached the end of his life. I want to comfort her, wrap my arms around her and tell her it will be alright, but of course I can't do that, for various reasons, but the main one is, I just don't know if her dog will be okay. I look down at George, who is watching the exit door intently. I have my own private battles to worry about right now, so I don't have the strength to console anyone else.

***

Suddenly the doors swing open and a young nurse walks towards us, shouting George's name as she does so. George immediately recognises her as his favourite nurse, Dani, who has cared for him over the past twelve months. He wags his tail wildly, his brown eyes light up with that familiar sparkle. Dani and George embrace lovingly and I notice other people in the waiting room smiling at the happy reunion. I smile too, grateful that just for a moment, sadness and worry disappear, as we watch our dog's obvious happiness as he greets his friendly nurse. For George at least, cancer is forgotten as he wraps himself around Dani's legs, looking for a treat no doubt. Sadly there is no treat as George heads off for a general anaesthetic and scans which will determine his immediate future. After a long hug with our lively Cavalier, we leave and I take a momentary glance back at him, to see him heading down the corridor to the theatre, wagging his tail and looking up at Dani without a care in the world.

We have decided to spend the time waiting for George in the local Ikea store which is just a few miles away. As

George will be in the hospital for quite a few hours, we have to distract ourselves from what we will be facing and the best way to do this is to get lost in Ikea. It really is possible to get lost in Ikea, but it is also a joy, as halfway round the store is the Swedish style restaurant and I can't resist having the meatballs for lunch. If there was ever a perfect comfort food, then it is Ikea meatballs with berry sauce and chips.

***

Walking round Ikea, eager to get to the restaurant, isn't that easy. The walkways are busy with people constantly stopping to view the furniture, glancing at lists of measurements on their phones.

'Do you think this sofa will fit, Theo?'

'Well, the only way to find out is to measure it.'

Theo proceeds to measure the aforementioned sofa and finally declares that the sofa is, in fact, too big.

'Nooo, Theo. Measure it again! I really want this sofa. Measure it with a different tape measure. Here, try this one.'

Theo takes the new tape measure from his beloved, rolling his eyes as he does so. He promptly measures the sofa once more, sighs and grimaces.

'I'm sorry Chloe but the measurements are the same. It won't fit. Let's look for another sofa.'

Chloe looks crestfallen and for a moment I am worried she might have a full blown tantrum. But no, she smiles sweetly, blinks rapidly and clears her throat.

'Well, do you think we should think about moving house Theo? Then we can get a big sofa.'

Theo takes on the appearance of a man who has just been asked the most difficult question in the world, in Latin. His face morphs into a ghostly white image, while his eyes take on a glassy, lost look of a young boy who is wondering if Father Christmas exists. Theo doesn't move, his body seemingly frozen in time.

'Theo, are you okay? THEO!'

Chloe grabs him by the arm and shakes him and he smiles at her, sighing as he does so.

'Chloe, why don't we go to the restaurant and get your favourite for lunch. Meatballs!'

Chloe smiles, and they head off in search of meatballs, hand in hand. Silently I congratulate Theo on a great choice of lunch, and on handling a difficult situation with calmness and dignity. My best guess is that he has used that technique before during one of Chloe's 'off the wall' suggestions. I am tempted to suggest that he can buy the frozen meatballs in the Ikea shop, just in case a similar situation arises at home.

***

I think of Theo and Chloe a few minutes later as I eat my own plate of delicious meatballs, and I make a note to visit the shop on my way out for my own supply at home. I finish my plate of ten meatballs and instantly want to eat them again, knowing deep down that I am full to bursting, so having seconds is vitually impossible right now.

It is mid afternoon as we are walking through the kitchen area of Ikea when my phone rings loudly. It is the veterinary hospital with news of George. As I stare at a shelf of various stainless steel cutlery, I hear the wonderful news that George is finally cancer free. The world stops for a moment and I think of all the sleepless nights, endless cuddles with George, frantically taking photos to make sure I have enough for my memory book. Is a thousand in one month too many, I ask myself? The call ends and I breathe again. We smile and turn 180 degrees heading back to the restaurant. There is only one way to celebrate. A cup of tea and a piece of Swedish chocolate cake. Anyway I've had enough of staring at furniture and homeware. My boy is going to be okay and I can't wait to see him for big cuddles and his favourite treat.

When we finally head out of Ikea to pick up George, we pass Theo and Chloe who are now looking at rather large plants in ceramic pots. I am praying for Theo's sake that the chosen plants are not so big that his beloved wants to move house again. I smile to myself as I see Theo selecting a small, delicate orchid and hands it to Chloe. She smiles and nods in agreement as she places the selected plant in the trolley. I have to hand it to Theo. He has style and tact. That young man will go far in life.

Arriving home at last with our beautiful, cancer free George, I fall into bed, ready for a restful sleep. It has been a good day. We have a healthy dog, my tummy is full after a delicious Ikea lunch and we have a freezer stocked full of meatballs.

***

Three things I am grateful for today.

1 Clever vets.

2 Ikea meatballs.

3 Theo and Chloe who made me smile today.

Chapter Twenty-Eight

Wednesday 18th October 2023

Today is the funeral of my dear friend Marilynne, although I still can't believe she is no longer here. I have known Marilynne for over fifty years and she was just 'always there.' Her sudden passing in September came as a shock, and here we are a few weeks later and I still can't grasp the enormity of it all, the final curtain, the last goodbye. I feel as though grief has been a constant throughout this year, my shadow, the black cloud suppressing my inner joy. And yet, the sun continues to shine, the rain still falls and the wind still howls its lamenting cry around my feet. Somehow grief attacks our inner soul, but we find the strength to carry on, regardless of the emptiness that punches through our heart.

I go to my wardrobe and pull out my 'funeral outfit'. You know the one. The one outfit we keep tucked away at the back of the wardrobe, praying we don't have to wear it any time soon. It hangs there, limp and lifeless, a black void, silent and yet holding so much power over me. I drape it over the wardrobe mirror. Memories of its last outing washing over me, overwhelming me, threatening to drown me. Was it really seven months ago that my black dress and I were joined in grief at Mum's funeral? I gently hold the soft fabric in my hands, caressing it, feeling for the last connection I had with her, on that sad day back in March. They say the real grief starts after the funeral, after the floral tributes have withered, and the sympathy cards have gathered dust on the window sill. Then reality hits, that you will never see that person again. I reluctantly put on the black dress, inwardly wishing I could rip it into shreds and burn it on a garden bonfire, resentful of what it represents.

As I sit in the car on the way to the church, I watch people getting on with their lives, oblivious to my discomfort and heartache right now. A young mother wearily pushes a pram up a steep hill, probably dreaming of a refreshing, hot cup of tea when she gets home, with her feet up, enjoying a peaceful five minutes. I hope she gets her peace. I remember those days of tiring motherhood duties and cold cups of tea that stood isolated on the coffee table, often never consumed.

I watch a postman dressed in pillar box red, whistling as he walks from door to door, posting letters and parcels. He looks happy and relaxed and I smile inwardly, glad that he enjoys his job. And yes, he has shorts on, even in this cool October weather. 'Life goes on' is a familiar saying and I am never sure if it is helpful to someone who is grieving. It is almost a dismissive statement, attempting to diminish the grief in some way. For myself, it never works. Yes, life does go on and the bereaved know that, but we just don't want to hear it, not yet anyway.

It is 5.30pm and I am back at home drinking a milky coffee. It has been a long emotional day and I just don't have the words right now to process it all. It all seems so final. The loss of a person in your life that you have known forever is difficult to accept. I am sat on the sofa eating comforting chocolate biscuits, whilst looking at old photos of Marilynne. I smile and gasp at a photo which was taken in the summer of 1986. I am heavily pregnant with my first child and Marilynne is attempting to fix the bow on the front of my dress. The image takes me by surprise as the details of that day are so clear, as though it happened yesterday. I remember the dress and the cream silk bow that tied at the front, the tiredness I was feeling, the anxiety at what was to come. Marilynne was a perfectionist and I remember her telling me that I hadn't tied the bow correctly. I was consumed with a 'couldn't care less' attitude, probably due to pregnancy fatigue, but she persisted in tying the bow correctly for me.

To this day, I still recall the feeling that she was doing everything she could to care for and nurture me, during what had been a difficult pregnancy, even down to the small detail of tying my bow correctly. How I wish she were here now so I could truly thank her for her kindness, but especially for ensuring that I looked my best that day, even though I wasn't feeling it. It is ironic that we only truly appreciate someone when they have gone. How I wish human nature was more aware of the preciousness of life, holding it close, scared to let it go in case it withers away at a moment's notice. But the reality is quite different, as people rush about their lives, ignoring the fragility of life and those closest to us. Isn't it time that we stopped the modern scourge of business and paused to appreciate all that we have?

Wherever you are Marilynne. Thank you for your friendship and thank you for tying my bow. Thank you for the years of fun, late night chats and sharing tears during difficult times in our lives. Thank you for your love of animals and especially for all the cuddles you gave George. I miss you already.

***

Three things I am grateful for today.

1 The gift of friendship.

2 My first born child.

3 Marilynne.

Chapter Twenty-Nine

Thursday 26th October 2023

Today we moved house. It was the most joyous and stressful moment all wrapped up together in one package, but we did it! I have felt unsettled for a few years, never quite feeling I am in the 'right place.' But, at last, I am standing in an empty lounge knowing that I am finally here. I am in the 'right place.' Of course, moving house is stressful, but the stress is productive, a sign you are finally getting somewhere, a step closer to where you belong – and I belong here. I am waiting for the removal van to arrive, a flask of tea in my hand and a sneaky bar of chocolate in my pocket. I am looking through a window with no curtains watching people walk by, maybe they are my new neighbours, maybe we will become friends? It feels like a new start to my life. So much has changed over the past year, that it seemed inevitable that a house move would complete the story. So here we go, our second house move in less than twelve months, but with the feeling that this house is a 'keeper.'

***

The removal van has arrived so the craziness begins. The first crazy thought comes from my husband who seems to be especially anxious about a particular packing box.

'So, which box has my tool box in it?'

Looking at a vast sea of brown cardboard packing boxes that all look the same, I smile sarcastically and shrug my shoulders.

'Take your pick.'

***

Yes, I know I am not very helpful, but my priority now is to find the box with the kettle and the chocolate biscuits. The toolbox can wait, quite honestly. It amazes me how men and women think differently about life issues. I tried for many years to get into the mind and thought processes of a man, but I honestly gave up. We really are from two different planets. I decide that I will do my version of moving house and my husband can do his version. Then we will both be happy. I will be content with my cup of tea and chocolate biscuits, and he will be happy with his tool box, drilling holes into walls to his heart's content. But what's the betting that any time soon he wants a cup of tea using boiled water from the kettle I have just unpacked. Kettle or tool box? No contest!

The removal men do a very efficient job, working quickly and silently, distributing all the boxes into the right room. I listen to them whistling merry tunes as they effortlessly lift heavy furniture through the house, with not one negative word among them. It is so reassuring to see someone else who loves their job. When someone is happy it is often contagious, and I feel a real spring in my step watching them work, singing as they go. The removal men enjoy an afternoon cup of tea with a plateful of chocolate biscuits sat in their van, resting their feet on the dashboard, still smiling, still happy. I bet they were very happy I found the box with the kettle in it!

***

My other half is still searching for his tool box and while I should be concerned about this, I don't feel any guilt about not helping him search. It's all about priorities you see, and I have just found the bedding box and I am proceeding up stairs to make up the bed for tonight. As I unfold the sheet I can hear him muttering under his breath in the next room.

'Why didn't I label these damn boxes?'

***

I can hear more mutterings as he rips open boxes rummaging through the contents like a man possessed. I am tempted, but I resist to tell him that all the boxes I packed were correctly labelled, which is why we now have a kettle and other essential kitchen items, and also why we will have a cosy bed tonight. I predict that we won't have a tool box by the end of the day, but as the saying goes, 'life goes on.'

It is nearly midnight and I am feeling rather tired, although happy. The house looks in disarray, except for the living room which has taken shape rather quickly, much to my husband's surprise who has spent most of his day lamenting the loss of his beloved tool box. We each take a sofa and put our feet up with a mug of coffee, courtesy of the kettle that I unpacked twelve hours ago!

***

'Well, we did it! Here we are at last. Our new home. Our new start. Are you happy?'

'Yes, I'm very happy....well...apart from...'

I look across at my husband, his face showing signs of weariness and yes, contentment.

'I just wanted to find my tool box and I am worried I have lost it.'

Sometimes as a wife, I have no words and there are times it is best to keep silent. Instead I give him a reassuring smile.

'Don't worry. We will find it tomorrow. Let's go to bed. It's been a long day and at least we have a bed ready made with new, fresh sheets on.'

***

As we head upstairs I quickly pop into the guest bedroom to check how many boxes are left to unpack and suddenly I spot the infamous tool box. It lies quietly and unassuming at the bottom of an already opened box. I smile to myself, wondering how my lovely husband has missed it, but equally I'm not surprised. I grab the offending tool box and run into the bedroom eager to show him my find. But all is quiet and there he lays in the newly made bed, already sleeping soundly, probably dreaming of his stressful day. I decide to leave him sleeping and I place the tool box in a prominent position next to the bed. It will be the first thing he sees on waking and I think tomorrow will be a happier and less stressed day for him.

I finally get into bed after a happy and successful house move, but quietly dreading the noise from drilling that will be taking over the house tomorrow. As I lay down on my soft, freshly laundered pillow, I pray I don't dream about tool boxes and unlabelled brown packing boxes. I suddenly realise that for the first time in a long time, there is a quiet peace resonating through my mind and body. I want to enjoy this moment for ever, so I decide against my usual overthinking and just accept that peace is finally here.

***

Three things to be grateful for today.

1 Finding the kettle within twenty minutes of looking.

2 A warm, safe place to live.

3 Finding the tool box and proving that girls always know best.

Chapter Thirty

Sunday 12th November 2023

My day starts with a walk along the river with my dog George. The sky holds dirty grey clouds and the air feels damp. I snuggle into my heavyweight winter coat as I watch George chase an insect, failing to catch it, of course. I never fail to notice the changes in seasons, but this year I have allowed myself to really engage in nature and its movement, as it goes from one month to another. As we are now firmly in Autumn, the riverbank takes on a different persona. At first glance it appears withered and dying, but as I look closer I can see life hidden in all the brown crispy plants which wrap around the river. Wildlife is busy preparing for winter and there is much work to be done before the cold, stark weather sets in. Chestnut brown leaves with hues of russet and chocolate crunch beneath my feet, triggering the child in me to laugh as I walk through them. Even now, as I look closer I can see tiny pea green buds on some of the trees. A sure sign that nature, like life, never stops turning and changing.

***

I meet a fellow dog walker who stops to talk, oblivious of our dogs who seem to have already started the usual bottom-sniffing ritual dance.

'Morning, I wouldn't go any further young lady. It's real muddy down there and you don't have any galoshes.'

I smile and suppress a slight giggle. I am flattered that the kind gentleman thinks I am young, but I am also amused by his use of the word 'galoshes.' My Mum also used the word galoshes instead of wellies and it always made me laugh.

I bid farewell to the gentleman and carry on down the path regardless of the warning, but I soon regret it. My hiking boots are no match for the deep, sticky mud that soon covers the pathway and I find myself stuck, my feet glued to the earth, my protestations go unheard.

'What did I tell you young lady? No galoshes!'

***

The gentleman soon becomes my knight in shining armour as he gently helps me release my muddy boots from the mud mire. We walk back together down a well trodden, but mud free path where he talks about the various wildlife that he often sees on his daily walk by the river. I am amazed at his knowledge and his generosity in sharing it with me and I wonder how much the younger generation would benefit from listening to their wiser elders. I suddenly think about my Mum and how many times I rebelled against her when she tried to give me advice. How I wish I had listened more. She had more wisdom than I ever appreciated. If only I had known that at the time.

Today is Remembrance Sunday in the UK when we remember all those British service members who have died in military conflicts. I stand at the Cenotaph in my local town with many others, red poppy pinned to my coat, head bowed in silence, lost in my own thoughts. Prayers are read and the two minute silence is observed and the crowd quietly disperses, having gently paid their respects to those that gave their life for freedom. I walk slowly behind a group of women who are comparing poppies on each other's coats.

***

'I do love your poppy Anne.'

'Thank you. I spent all last week crocheting it. It's slightly different from last years. I wanted a bigger one this year.'

'Well, it's lovely Anne. Do you like mine? I made it out of an old velvet dress I hadn't worn for ages.'

'Ooh, clever you. It's very nice.'

***

I glance down at my own red poppy. A solitary, simple poppy, that I made myself last week, using some left over red organza I found in my craft drawer. I wonder if I could find some red velvet for next year and make a new brooch. I do think I will be crafting more next year as I find it relaxing and a way to escape from the sad thoughts.

This afternoon I spend relaxing at home and decide to watch a classic film, snuggled on the sofa. The film of choice is The Great Escape which is one of my favourites. As the film finishes I think of all those who fought in the wars to ensure peace. I wonder if we truly know and understand just how much they sacrificed in order to achieve this peace. My Mum was only ten when the Second World War broke out. I wonder if she was scared hearing the news. I wonder how she felt hearing the air raid sirens and rushing to the shelters, as the threat of bombing loomed. I wish I had talked to her more about her memories of the War, so I could grasp the enormity of the situation that she found herself in. I wonder if this is a normal part of grief? Regretting things not said, places not visited, opportunities not taken. I do find myself saying 'I wish....' many times when I am thinking about Mum. I need to stop it. It's not useful or helpful.

I am awake most of the night thinking about the wars and the people that were affected by them. I snuggle down in my cosy bed, feeling safe and protected and I know that I am very lucky and privileged. It's the little things like this that I am thinking about more this year. Grief does that. It makes you take notice of the things you never noticed before. I vow to always notice the little things, to be grateful of all I have. I also make a promise to myself that I will never take those that I love for granted. I am feeling blessed and grateful tonight, very grateful. I really miss Mum but was so thankful to have her in my life.

***

Three things I am grateful for today.

1 Those that fought in the wars to save the country from tyranny.

2 Galoshes (or wellies) for rainy and muddy days – even though I didn't wear them today when I really needed them.

3 Steve McQueen in the film 'The Great Escape.' He cheered up my Sunday afternoon.

Chapter Thirty-One

Saturday 18th November 2023

Pulling the curtains back on a new day, I can see a hint of blue sky peeking through the clouds. One of my dearest friends, Niki, is on her way to my house, and together we will be visiting the Knitting and Stitching Show, which is an annual event in my local town. My friend and I are both avid crafters and the thought of spending a day amongst a multitude of luscious fabrics and a rainbow of wool makes me very happy. I have enrolled on some mini workshops to learn new crafting techniques, including patchwork, which has me thinking that maybe now I can use that huge box of surplus fabric that is haunting me from the spare bedroom.

Linking arms, giggling like schoolgirls, Niki and I head into the main exhibition hall, where we stop to show our entry ticket. Except, we seem to have mislaid our tickets. There is a brief moment of concern, even panic, but then we smile at each other, eyes twinkling, knowing that even this slight problem will probably be overcome. Niki and I have been friends for over twenty five years and have experienced many mishaps and adventures together. We have the same philosophy in life. Panic, smile, then find a solution. It works, as it always does and a few minutes later, we enter the first exhibition hall, stopping to take in the view before us.

The exhibition hall is literally buzzing with excitement. Ladies and gentlemen of all ages are moving around the different stalls and stands, laden with bags of their crafty purchases. The atmosphere is infectious and I can feel my credit card warming up in my bag, anticipating its use. We head for the fabric stalls, a cornucopia of shiny textiles in every possible design you could think of. Each roll of material longing to be touched and caressed. Hundreds of people moving in harmony, admiring every offering of fabric on each stall.

***

Feel this, Jill. It's heavenly. I must make my Christmas dress from this.'

'Oh, this design is just exquisite. The detailing on the flowers is like an oil painting. Four metres please!'

'Excuse me please. I saw this fabric first and it is for a special occasion. My Mother of the Bride outfit.'

'Do you think red suits me, Ellen? Does it make me look like a tart?'

'I shouldn't really. I've already spent over £100. Oh, go on then. Give me five metres of this.'

'This fabric will make a wonderful summer dress. Do you think we will have a summer next year? Probably not.'

'I'm not really a dressmaker, but this fabric is too gorgeous to leave. Three metres please.'

***

And so it goes on (the last one was me, by the way.)

Eager crafters and dressmakers enjoying a day of spending, chatting and learning new crafts, excited at what else lies around the corner. What strikes me is the friendship between all the visitors, most of them strangers to each other. All joined together with a common love of crafts, members of the same club, all with a silent understanding of the emotions and feelings that come with this exclusive membership.

I move on to the workshop I have booked, English patchwork. I am such a beginner that I didn't even know English patchwork was a thing. But within five minutes of joining the workshop, I learn very quickly that there are many different forms of patchwork. I sit next to a young woman who has travelled some distance to be at the workshop today. We talk about our love of learning new crafts, and I ask her why she loves crafting so much. She gently explains that she has been suffering from chronic anxiety, and crafting helps her to relax. She tells me she enjoys embroidery and likens it to meditation, explaining that she becomes so engrossed in creating art with colourful stitches, that her anxiety disappears.

I listen to the patchwork teacher, but in the back of my mind I think about the young woman and her embroidery. My thoughts drift, as I wonder if crafting should be a therapy prescribed by the NHS for anxious and depressed patients. Surely the joy of creating something special with your own hands must outweigh the trauma of taking prescription drugs, which only mask the problem anyway. I conclude that the world would be a better place if we all became more creative and mindful about what we do.

I finish the workshop with a tiny piece of completed patchwork, measuring about six inches square, and mentally note that my dream of creating a patchwork bed cover may take longer than expected. Grasping my precious piece of patchwork, I head back into the main hall and the first trade stall I see is laden with embroidery products. For a second I stop in my tracks. I think back to the recent conversation with my workshop companion. This feels like fate. My anxiety levels have been super high since Mum passed away, so maybe I would benefit from embroidery myself. I fill a shopping bag with soft, tactile threads, embroidery hoops, needles and template patterns. My dream of creating a patchwork quilt by Christmas is long gone.

***

My friend and I meet up for coffee and cake and I notice we need two extra chairs for our bags of all our purchases. We giggle as we eat lemon drizzle cake, knowing we have seriously overspent today, but laughing because we honestly don't care. We are enjoying ourselves among other creatives and it feels good. I make a mental note that sometimes 'money DOES bring you happiness.' We sit on a communal table which is busy right now. Looks like everyone is on 'coffee and cake' mode. An elderly couple sit next to us, husband and wife I presume.

'Are you having a good day, Bea?'

'Oh, yes, Patrick. I really am. Isn't it wonderful? I have so many new crafts to start when I get home. I'm so excited.'

I'm so glad you are having a good day. I love to see you smile.'

'Thank you for buying me all these wonderful things today.'

'That's okay dear. I love you.'

***

Leaving the lovebirds to eat their cake, I feel a huge warm rush all over my body. In the middle of the chaos of the show, I have learnt that crafting can help with anxiety and I have also learnt that love still exists, even after spending a huge amount of money from the joint bank account. Dragging my bulging bags back to my car, I keep this thought close to the forefront of my mind, and hope beyond hope that my husband sees it the same way, when he becomes aware of how much I have spent. Or maybe it's easier not to mention it. I could just leave my bags in the car for now, couldn't I?

***

Three things to be grateful for today.

1 Crafting. A great healer and soother of tired minds.

2 Like minded people who understand my passion for my hobbies.

3 My friend Niki for never failing to make me laugh. Everyone should have a 'Niki' in their lives.

PS. I am enjoying learning embroidery and yes, it really does help lessen anxiety. Thank you to my workshop friend for the advice.

Chapter Thirty-Two

Tuesday 19th December 2023

Christmas is nearly here. I have mixed feelings about it. My first Christmas without Mum brings apprehension, interspersed with sadness. Yesterday I cried at the sight of fairy lights glistening in local streets, heralding the coming of the festive season. Today I am in town buying last minute gifts, but distracted by thoughts of Mum. I feel drawn into Marks and Spencer to buy her a warm fleecy dressing gown, as I did every year. And so, I find myself in the nightwear department, looking, but with no one to buy for. Those days of fleece dressing gowns are gone, my head knows it, but my heart is still playing catch up. I knew my first Christmas without her would be difficult, but I never imagined the sight of a fleece dressing gown would bring tears to my eyes. Inwardly, I say to myself that this is just a process, a path I must walk on in order to get to the other side. Even so, I cast my eyes on the dressing gowns once more and come to the conclusion that Mum would definitely have picked the pale pink one. Some habits are hard to release and I remind myself that I am not perfect.

***

I smile at the sight of a man, about my age, also eyeing up the dressing gowns. He is smartly dressed in a long black wool coat, his neck wears a red cashmere scarf. He looks a little awkward. Maybe he has lost his mother too. Suddenly he is joined by a small, elegant lady of about eighty years old. She too is dressed very smartly, with an air of French chic, a silk scarf adorns her neckline.

'What about this one Mother?' Mr 'Red Cashmere Scarf' strokes a soft pink dressing gown, while checking the price tag.

'Oh Robert dear. It looks like a hospital dressing gown. Try be more classy.'

'Mother, must we go through this every year?' Why don't you let me choose your present? Then I can surprise you.'

'Robert, you know how I hate surprises, which is why I like to choose my own dressing gown. And anyhow, I don't like your style'

Robert looks crestfallen. He knows his sense of fashion deserted him many years ago, but he probably didn't expect his own mother to attack his lack of style.

***

I watch mother and son walking round and round in circles, trying to draw the Christmas present problem to a conclusion. It doesn't happen quickly and I leave them to their dilemma.

Later that evening I am sat inside a church, wrapped in a warm wool cape to try combat the icy weather, while attempting to look a little stylish. I am here for a carol concert, along with many other people, who also appear to be dressed for the festive occasion. The church is beautifully lit by candles, projecting a feeling of peace, with hundreds of twinkling lights creating an almost fairylike atmosphere. I am hypnotised by the lights as they dance and sway and I suddenly feel calm. Mum would have loved it here, the carols, the solo singers, the mince pies and fruit punch served afterwards. In a funny way, I almost feel her presence, drifting in and out, her spirit holding me close. My body warms and glows from within, so much so, that I have to remove my cape for fear of becoming too warm. I grapple with the large voluminous cape, trying to remove it without disturbing the lady sat next to me. I fail miserably and manage to knock her elegant hat from her head. I watch in shame as the hat falls to the ground and rolls under the chair in front of her. I am mortified but she laughs. I sit back in my chair, relieved that she finds it humorous.

I suddenly become aware that the calmness I experienced earlier seems to have spread throughout the rest of the congregation. It isn't just my hatless lady that projects calm, the room is also calm. I'm not sure if it's the atmosphere of the candles and church together, or if it's the fruit punch that was served on arrival, but there is a serenity in the church that envelopes me. Is this finally peace in my heart I am feeling? I hold my breath, not wanting to let it go, whatever it is.

People are smiling, exchanging hugs, helping older ones to their seats, sharing carol sheets, and just generally taking care of each other. In the blink of an eye, strangers become friends and age barriers are dropped. As the carols start I feel a strange sense of belonging to the world that I left following my Mum's passing in February. I feel like I am on my way back. I'm not sure where I've been, but I am singing with a heart full to bursting. I'm not particularly religious, but I do feel a sense of being cared for and held safely – by what or who, I'm not sure. The concert passes in a blur, while I'm still trying to compute how I feel.

Following the concert we retire to the back of church for more fruit punch and mince pies. The strong sense of community continues, as complete strangers engage me in conversation, and I am embraced with genuine affection. I have always rallied against the false meaning of Christmas, with all the trappings of 21st century materialism, but tonight has brought me closer to a 'real' Christmas. I return home with a real feeling of joy filling my whole being. I know that this Christmas will be difficult without Mum, but for now, I'm just going to be grateful for all I have.

***

Three things I am grateful for today.

1 Christmas Carol concerts.

2 My black cape that keeps me warm.

3 Fluffy dressing gowns from Marks and Spencer. Thank you for keeping my Mum warm every winter.

Chapter Thirty-Three

Monday 25th December 2023

Happy Christmas to me. My first Christmas without Mum, the day I had been dreading, to be honest. The day starts quiet with a walk across the fields with George, our dog. The air feels crisp and I am glad it isn't raining as we trek across open land. We meet a multitude of other walkers on our journey, some alone and some with families. I wonder about everyone's circumstances and how they will spend the day.

***

A family of three generations walk just ahead of us. Young children squeal as they play chase with their grandad while their grandmother tells them all to be careful (isn't that what all grandmothers do?). The parents of the children walk slower than the rest of the group, and I deduce that they are trying to enjoy a few moments peace away from their responsibility as parents. I find it reassuring to watch them. Generations of families still able to come together to celebrate Christmas, even as the world progresses at such a fast rate. As the walk takes a steep incline, the grandparents of the family group drop back to walk just in front of us, allowing the parents to take over the supervision of the children.

'Baileys tonight, Jane?'

'Oh yes, Baileys, and maybe we can open that box of chocolates the kids got us?'

The family head off into the distance, and I notice the grandparents holding hands as they climb the hill, pulling each other up the more difficult parts. I quietly hope they have a lovely Christmas Day, followed by a Baileys and a chocolate or two.

***

We walk for another thirty minutes before heading home to dinner and feet up in front of the TV. If I am honest, I almost want the day to be over quickly. We are having a quiet day and eating Christmas dinner alone, as family have committments elsewhere. Except, we are not actually having Christmas dinner as I couldn't face it, so it looks like a pizza is on the cards, which suits me fine. I can see White Christmas is on TV, which is one of my favourite films, so I will be happy singing along with Bing Crosby later this afternoon.

The day is passing by quickly, fueled by the usual Christmas TV offerings and copious amounts of Terry's Chocolate Orange segments. I do spend some of the time reflecting on the past and lapsing into memories of spending Christmas Day with Mum and Dad. I sometimes lament the changes in the world as life seemed so simple forty years ago, just before I had my children. But as in all historical eras, time does move on and things change. I know 2023 has been a year of great change for me, and I have honestly struggled to move with the times. I have punished myself for grieving, for not being able to move on, but now I see that grieving is so different for each individual. Who actually sets the rules for grieving? Who says we have to grieve a certain way or for a certain length time? The answer is, no one!

As the year closes in, I feel I have learnt so much and developed in ways I never thought possible. Christmas is just a catalyst when things seem to come together, when people sit and think about what is truly important to them. I am no different. As I turn the Christmas lights off and head up to bed, I think of all those grieving tonight, their loved ones, our friends and family. I hope that they can find comfort in something, even just a little thing, just something that brings a flash of joy, just for a moment. It has been an emotional day, but I got there in the end, as I always do.

Goodnight Christmas 2023.

***

Three things I am grateful for today.

1 Family and friends that wished me Happy Christmas today.

2 Bing Crosby singing White Christmas.

3 Terry's Chocolate Orange – there is nothing like it.

Chapter Thirty-Four

Monday 22nd January 2024

January is often known as 'The Blue Month' as most people feel a genuine sadness and low mood during this time. Unfortunately I am no exception. The positivity of December has floated away on the cold wind of winter, and I am feeling isolated and unsure what this year will bring. The oncoming anniversary of Mum's passing next month is also playing on my mind, with the sudden realisation that it is nearly twelve months since I saw her or spoke to her. That thought sends me into a spiralling panic, as I feel I still have so much to say to her, so much news to catch up on, and I just want to see her lovely face.

January has brought a myriad of health issues too. Maybe it's the damp weather, or the overall feeling of gloom that lies heavy in the air. But every day I take one step forward, looking for those joyful moments in life that often pass us by if we don't look for them. Today I am in the opticians, waiting for an eye test. I know for sure that my eyes have changed. Old age, I reckon. The optician never actually says it, but I know she is thinking it. I am even eligible for a free eye test now I am sixty. Go me! The excitement of getting something for free is unbearable. I am joking, of course. The waiting room is busy and I have forgotten my book to read. I sigh.

***

I am sat opposite a woman of about forty years old, who is talking quietly to her young son, aged about seven. There is obviously some tension between them as the young boy is sat with his arms tightly folded, glaring into the space in front of him. The silence is abruptly ended.

'I just want Spiderman glasses, Mummy,'

Ten minutes later I watch them leave, the young boy proudly wearing a brightly coloured pair of red rimmed spectacles, AKA Spiderman. His mother looks happy, probably relieved that a major crisis has been averted. After all who wants to argue with Spideman?

***

I sit in the consulting room getting my eyes tested, a process I dislike intensely. I always feel that I am not completing the tests correctly. I squint and blink rapidly, in the hope that I finish the testing with flying colours. I'm not sure why I do that. After all, there is no gold star if you pass the tests, only a huge bill waiting for you, as you choose yet more new spectacles.

The testing is finished, and I am downstairs looking for a new pair of glasses, with a quivering credit card in my hand. I wander round aimlessly, hoping inspiration will jump out at me. It rarely does. How can a person choose a new pair of spectacles when we can't see properly in the first place? It's a mystery, to be honest. Thankfully I am not alone with my thoughts.

***

A young woman stands next to me admiring the latest Kylie Minogue designer frames. She leans forward, squinting and frowning simultaneously. She reaches for a tortoiseshell design (at least I think it is tortoiseshell) and pops them on, looking in the mirror as she does so. She moves closer to the mirror, pulling faces and tilting her head. Suddenly she turns to me and smiles.

'Excuse me. Do you think these suit me? I'm not sure and I can't see very well.'

I move a little closer, as I too can't see clearly.

'Yes, they look great on you. A good choice!'

She smiles broadly and thanks me. To be honest it was just a wild guess as I was struggling to see them myself, without getting too close to her. Oh, the joys of being short sighted.

***

I manage to buy some new spectacles for myself, reverting back to a similar pair I once had. The stress of trying to choose new glasses overwhelms me and I opt for the easy way out. Cowardly, I know, but necessary.

It is early evening and I am out walking George, our dog. The air is cool and bites through me, numbing my extremities, chilling my cheeks. George is oblivious to the Yorkshire winter weather, preferring to direct his thoughts onto more important matters, like which dog walked this path before me? And how many times did he pee against this tree? I come to the conclusion that humans think too much. We analyse every word and action of every other human being, until our head hurts thinking about it all. We retain sad thoughts until our heart breaks. We can't let go of hurtful things that were said to us years ago. We ruminate and chew every negative word, and yet, we still refuse to spit it out. My relationship with grief has been the same. I find myself rehashing every detail of Mum's death, trying to find a way through it that will make me feel better. I have been trying for nearly a year, and yet my thoughts have remained stagnant. I watch George, walking carefree, accepting the world for what it is, in this present moment and then suddenly, a light bulb switches on in my head, causing me to stop abruptly. I need to let go. I need to accept. I need to live for now, the present moment. Mum would want me to do that. 'Be more like George.' I can hear her say.

The winter darkness closes in, the biting wind catches my breath and George and I head home. I am noticeably warmer as I walk through the deserted streets, the moonlight guiding me home. One final look at the stars as I close the door. Goodnight Mum, wherever you are. I miss you.

***

Three things I am grateful for today.

1 Opticians to help us look after our eyes.

2 Spiderman glasses that make children happy.

3 The moonlight to help us see our way through the darkness.

Chapter Thirty-Five

Monday 29th January 2024

Another day, another health issue, but this one is a little more of a worry. Just after Mum's passing, I started having chest pains. I put them down to stress, but as time went on I knew I couldn't ignore them anymore. And so, I find myself at the doctors surgery waiting to have a heart monitor fitted for twenty four hours. The stress of waiting is actually sending my heart rate rocketing. I can feel it in my chest, my breathing shallow and fast. Can you imagine actually having a racing heart rate due to waiting for the heart monitor to be fitted, to check if you have indeed got a heart problem? I smile at the irony. My heart continues to pump through my chest, so I look round the room trying to find something to occupy my mind, to distract myself from the issue.

An elderly gentleman sits opposite me and he too is gazing round the room. Our eyes lock for a moment, and we nod and smile together, acknowledging that we both are feeling anxious right now. I wonder what he is worried about. I know he can't be having a heart monitor fitted, as the surgery only has one, and today is my lucky day. I hope it's nothing too serious for him.

A door opens and I hear my name being called. I reluctantly drag myself from the chair, smiling at the elderly gentleman, and I enter a small room at the back of the surgery. A bright young medical assistant explains what she will be doing to attach the heart monitor and I smile to let her know I understand, but in reality I would rather be at home having a cup of tea. My wish comes true and thirty minutes later I am at home comforting myself with Yorkshire Tea and a slice of cake. I personally think I deserve it. It's been a stressful day and it's only 10.30am.

My instructions are to act normal while wearing the monitor, but my instinct is to lie here all day, in the hope that no unusual readings are discovered. Of course, I realise this is unhelpful, so I get up from the sofa and start my day with my ever present friendly heart monitor following my every move. I run up the stairs looking for something I have mislaid and instantly regret it. I feel a little breathless. Is this due to my lack of fitness or something more sinister? I sneak a look at the monitor hoping it will give me a clue, a warning sign, but it is silent. I half expect an alarm to sound or a bright red light to flash violently, indicating danger, but there is nothing. I'm not sure if this is good news.

I decide to go to the gym to see if that will have an effect on the reading. I feel brave as I step on the crosstrainer, watching my heart rate increase on my watch. The elusive red warning light on the monitor still evades me, even though I try to incite it on the rowing machine and on the treadmill. Exhausted, I decide to go for a coffee to assess the last hour and my attempts to intimidate the dreaded heart monitor.

I perch on a comfy sofa drinking a welcome milky coffee, that comforts my confused mind and aching bones. A couple sit opposite me, also drinking coffee, while talking seriously to each other.

***

I've had a good day today, Janet. I've had a swim, been in the sauna and now I'm drinking a coffee.'

'I told you everything would be okay, didnt I?'

'Yes, but I thought I was a goner there, love. But here I am, large as life.'

***

I watch them as they both laugh, a genuine, happy laugh. I don't know what has happened, but my initial thought is that he has been given a second chance at life. I run my hand over the heart monitor, grateful that my heart still beats, whatever stress I put it through. I have a sudden thought that everything will be okay, my heart and my life, yes, even life without Mum. As humans, we come through the most extraordinary difficulties, we breathe and we move on. I am acutely aware that time is creeping up to the first anniversary of Mum's passing. I am determined that I will reach her anniversary, feeling considerably better than I did a year ago. My heart has been broken, but it is repairing itself slowly, even without the heart monitor that is currently stuck to my chest. The heart is a wonderful thing. It breaks, it repairs, it heals and life goes on. I get into bed with my monitor, hoping its presence doesn't give me bad dreams. Goodnight little heart monitor. Thank you for looking after me.

PS – Two weeks later I receive the results of the heart monitor from my doctor. Nothing abnormal detected. Thank you dear heart.

***

Three things I am grateful for today.

1 The NHS lending me a heart monitor to check my heart is working well.

2 A stranger for reminding me that sometimes we are given a second chance and we should grab it with both hands.

3 My heart – for giving me 60 years of wonderful service, for not breaking completely and for gently healing when I needed it the most.

Chapter Thirty-Six

Tuesday 20th February 2024

So here we are. The first year anniversary of Mum's passing. A day I have dreaded, but to be honest, now it is here, I am glad. It feels like an achievement to have reached this day without fearing I am going to crumble into tiny pieces and never recover. Today is all about Mum and celebrating her life, but it is also about grief and how I have coped, managed and got through it. Go me!

The grief experts say the first year is the most difficult for those left behind, a time of acceptance and readjustment, a time of wondering how you will manage without your loved one in your life. And yes, it was difficult. At times it was unbearable, but the days go by and somehow those days turn into months, and you find yourself another year on. Sometimes it feels surreal, as you live in a dream-like state, just doing enough to let the clock tick by on yet another grief ridden day. And yet, through journalling, I have found many genuine moments of joy. I have being swept away by intense feelings of gratitude, for my own life, yes, even on days where the grief bit hard and deep.

So today I find myself sat on a beach in Bridlington. I am holding a tiny amount of my beloved mother's ashes in a small wooden box that I deliberately kept back so I would have enough to scatter on her favourite beach. My fingers naturally caress the box, feeling every corner, every detail, infusing love through my hands deep into the ashes contained within. She is with me as I sit on the golden sand looking out to the grey North Sea, as it tumbles its way to the shoreline. It is an unexpected day of wall to wall sunshine and blue skies. Divine intervention perhaps? The weather certainly makes my difficult day easier and lighter.

The February sun warms my face which I tilt towards the sky. I want to drink the warm nectar of that big yellow ball, as it heals my anxious body of sadness. I feel immobile as I sit alone, quietly, gently, on this vast Yorkshire beach. I feel as though the beach has cleared just for this moment. Just me and Mum, and the sea, ready to accept Mum in a cloud of dust, to finally take her home, but still living within my heart.

I am nervous, yet determined that this is the right thing to do. Bridlington beach – the place of many family holidays, the place where my Mum taught my children how to build sandcastles, the place where she was happy watching her beloved grandchildren play freely without a care in the world. I am suddenly aware of my own precious memories as they trickle down my face in the guise of tears. I will never forget you Mum. Never.

I breathe deeply hoping for a sign that it is the right time. A seagull's cry, perhaps? A cloud in the shape of a heart? Wide eyed, I look intently, but no sign appears. I guess this is the moment that only I can decide. I take out my phone and take a photograph of the scene before me. I never want to forget this moment. Running my hand through the fine sand, I think of time and how it goes so quickly. It feels like yesterday I was sat on this very spot, with Mum and Dad and my young daughters, and now I am here alone to scatter my Mum's ashes, to say goodbye, one final time.

Brushing the sand away I make my way to the sea, clutching my precious box close to my chest. I hear only the roar of the waves as they crash on the shore, the wind as it sweeps across the bay. For a moment I feel totally isolated, alone in the world, now an orphan, devoid of parents and the feeling of security that they bring. I glance round and there is no one on the beach, except for a lone dog walker who is concentrating hard on throwing a ball for her four legged friend. I suddenly wish I wasn't alone. I have a momentary panic which subsides quickly, as I realise it has to be this way. It was just me and Mum at the beginning of my life, and now it is just me and Mum at the end of her journey.

As I spot sunbeams radiating from the bright sun I nod my head, acknowledging that it is now time. Yes, Mum. It is now time to say goodbye again. But this time we are not in some soulless crematorium. We are here together on the beach of memories where we spent so many happy times. I remove my shoes and wade out into the ice cold sea, waves gathering momentum around my frozen legs. I open the lid of the box and say 'I love you' as I tip it on its side, ready for the waves to catch the contents. At that moment a strong gust of wind blows in from nowhere and the dust scatters in the air, almost looking for a way to heaven. I grimace at the sandpaper texture on my lips. I smile. I take a deep breath. It is time for me to go. Back to reality. Back to my husband and my dog who are waiting on the harbour.

***

'How did it go love? OK?' Did you scatter the ashes OK?'

I smile. I laugh out loud. It could only happen to me!

'It went well, but I think I just ate Mum.'

Is it just me and my overactive imagination? But did I just hear Mum laughing somewhere in the ether?

***

Three things I am grateful for today.

1 Bridlington beach and the memories.

2 The Yorkshire sun. I needed to feel you today.

3 The unpredictable weather in Yorkshire. Mum would have laughed. Maybe she arranged it?

Chapter Thirty-Seven

Tuesday 27th February 2024

Today is my birthday. Happy Birthday to Me! I have come full circle on my journey through grief. Of course, my journey is not over. I don't believe you just stop grieving. I believe you learn to live with the grief. So this is not the end of my journey, but this is the end of documenting and journelling this important, and sometimes difficult first year.

So what have I learnt on this incredible and often sad journey? I have learnt that grief does not follow a set pattern and that for every individual, grief is a different experience. There is no rigid timeline or blueprint you need to follow. Grief just happens. We all have to do what we have to do, to get through each day. Yes, we can listen to others' experiences and we can read books and we can join support groups, but the grief is ours and ours alone. We each have our own path to walk along, and sometimes it can be lonely and isolated. We can lean on others for support, but at the end of each day as the night draws those dark curtains, we retire to our bed with our own thoughts, our own tears.

However, I quickly came to the conclusion that finding the little pockets of joy in each day can truly help us through the difficult times. As a writer and journalling teacher, I found it easy to document my daily observations of ordinary life. It is these observations that I found the most profound and comforting. Life goes on in so many ways. People walk their dogs, go to the dentist, eat fish and chips and drink coffee. All these so called ordinary events gave me so much joy, along with a feeling of 'life goes on.'

Since the passing of Mum I have felt a stronger desire to open my eyes and really observe what is going on around me. I started the process to help divert my attention from the pain I was feeling at losing Mum, but the process quickly turned into a daily longing for me, as I sought comfort in the 'little things.' I noticed the full colour spectrum of nature, the cornucopia of the noises of wildlife, the dance of flowers as they bloomed in the spring. As I journalled in my first year of grief, I became more self aware of my place in the world, and how I fitted in to my environment. I sought validation of my quirky habits and I received that validation. It was truly okay for me to stay in and read a book quietly, if that's what my heart wanted. If I wanted to sit in a field and watch lambs play freely, filling me with joy, then that was okay too. I viewed the world with awe and wonderment every day, rather than rushing through, missing all the joyous moments that generally pass us by. Expressing gratitude became routine for me and I honestly could not go through a day without finding something to be grateful for. It really helps to write down these thoughts of gratitude. Writing somehow validates the feelings. Why not try it yourself and notice the feeling of happiness that comes from it?

And so, this year of grief and gratitude comes to an end. My life goes on without Mum, but in a different way. I found a new me. Yes, a 'me' without Mum, but a 'me' she would be proud of. As I finish this book, I look out of the window. The sun is shining in a clear blue sky and I can see fluffy clouds floating gently across my view. I sometimes think of Mum perched on one of those clouds, drifting aimlessly but yet, stopping for a moment to wave and say hello to me.

I am still here, living in a beautiful world and so grateful for all I have, all I have experienced, and all I will experience in days and years to come. I hope you have enjoyed the journey with me, and I pray that if you too are going through grief, you somehow find a way through your difficult journey. And remember, there is always, ALWAYS something to be grateful for.

About The Author

Susanna lives in North Yorkshire and is an award winning writer, poet and author. She enjoys writing across all genres, including memoir, poetry, journalling, short stories, theatre plays, magazine / newspaper articles and novels, with a particular interest in cosy crime and whodunnits!

She is a trained therapeutic writing teacher, encouraging people of all ages and backgrounds to use the power of creative writing to improve health and wellbeing. Susanna has taught writing for wellbeing in schools, community groups, retirement groups and care homes and is passionate about supporting people to explore their own writing journey.

Susanna regularly holds online and in person workshops and classes in writing related topics.

In her spare time she enjoys rambling around the Yorkshire countryside with her dog George, exploring historic sites, photography, reading, getting lost in bookshops (much to her husband's consternation) and spending time with her family.

For more information on Susanna and her work, please visit – www.susannalewis.co.uk

Thank You

Writing a book can be a lonely and solitary activity, but this book would never have reached publication without the support of others. And so, I would like to thank the following people for their love, support and patience. Yes, patience! Especially during those moments of indecision about titles and bookcovers that all authors grapple with.

Firstly I would like to thank my husband Tony for his love and support. I am not an easy person to live with when I get tired due to a late night stint of writing, or when my laptop freezes and I am tempted to throw it out of the window!

To my three daughters, Sarah, Sophie and Rosie who gave me valuable input during the writing of this book and helped me focus on what was truly important.

To my dearest writing friends Cat, Gemma, Simon and Dave, whose support, love and encouragement was much needed and appreciated. Thank you for your writing expertise, advice and emotional support, helping me manage such a difficult topic to write about.

To Grace and my Joy Club friends. Your writing inspires me every day and I am lucky to be in the company of such wonderful creatives.

To Kate for advising me on writing a memoir following my Mum's passing. I took your wise advice and I hope you like this book.

To my non-writing friends who provided me with distractions, laughter and support when the pressure of writing became too much. Those breaks away from the screen were often the reason I persisted with my writing.

Finally my biggest thanks go to my beloved Mum. You always encouraged me to write and just before you passed away, you told me to carry on writing and not to waste my gift. I wish you were here to see this book, so I could say thank you in person. I hope I have done you proud Mum. I miss you and will love you forever.